CW00763181

HEART MASTER TRIPLE HEATER

MONKEY PRESS is named after the Monkey King in The Journey to the West, the 16th century classical novel by Wu Chengen. Monkey blends skill, initiative and wisdom with the spirit of freedom, irreverence and mischief.

AcuMedic CENTRE
101-105 CAMDEN HIGH STREET
LONDON NW1 7JN
Tel: 020 7388-6704/5783
info@acumedic.com   www.acumedic.com

HEART MASTER TRIPLE HEATER

Claude Larre and Elisabeth Rochat de la Vallée

transcribed and edited by Caroline Root

MONKEY PRESS

© Monkey Press 1992 Re-edited 1998
CHINESE MEDICINE FROM THE CLASSICS:
HEART MASTER TRIPLE HEATER
Claude Larre and Elisabeth Rochat de la Vallée

ISBN 1 872468 05 5

Text Editor: Caroline Root
Production and Design: Sandra Hill
Calligraphy: Qu Lei Lei

Printed on recycled paper by Spider Web, London

CONTENTS

All Nan jing illustrations are from the16th century commentary by Zhang Shixian.

FOREWORD

Six years have passed since the first edition of this book was published. These years have seen momentous developments within the profession of Oriental medicine in Great Britain. Most notable has been the creation of the British Acupuncture Council, which, like the European Community, brings in its wake a harmonization and a rationalization of standards. The British Acupuncture Accreditation Board and the Common Core Curriculum are now established, and determine, in part at least, the future of student education and the practice of acupunture in this country. It is therefore essential that voices distinct from the mainstream, and unaffected by the need to be 'on message' should be heard. Such voices are found in the work of Claude Larre s.j. and Elisabeth Rochat de la Vallee. Their perceptive insights into Chinese medicine past and present are invaluable, and unique in today's climate.

This book, concentrating as it does on the paired *zangfu* of the heart master and the triple heater, is rich in thought-provoking observations, detailed classical references and the teachers' usual blend of illuminating humour. The complexity and subtlety of these two energetic systems has rarely been explained and elucidated so well. The manifestation of the heart's active double aspect as *xin zhu* and *zin bao luo*, and the relation of the triple heater to the kidneys, fire and water, are all examined in detail and presented with elegance and precision.

This edition of the transcript of a seminar given in 1986, organized by Peter Firebrace for The International Register of Oriental Medicine, has been reedited to enhance the text's clarity, and Chinese characters have been included in the body of the text.

Caroline Root
Cambridge 1998

HEART MASTER

xin zhu

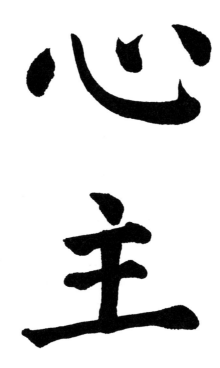

Xin zhu

HEART MASTER

Peter Firebrace: I would like to welcome Father Larre and Elisabeth to another seminar, the fourth in our series on the *zang fu.* It was about a year ago that we held our first one which covered Su wen chapter 8 with its concise descriptions of the twelve charges. In the last couple of seminars we have gone into much greater detail on each organ in turn, looking at their functions and movements, their harmony and disharmony, trying to understand how these concepts arise directly from the philosophical roots of Chinese medicine.

In the last seminar we covered the heart, in particular its more refined spiritual aspects and its relation with the spirits. This time we will start with the heart's more active aspect, *xin zhu* (心 主), and with related terms such as *xin bao luo* (心 包 絡), and then continue with a discussion of the triple heater.

Claude Larre: After these few words from Peter let us turn to Elisabeth to present the programme. It is not a good idea to have two presentations of the same thing if we are unsure whether the two spirits and two hearts see the main themes in the same manner! So for clarity's sake I propose that Elisabeth starts by telling you how she will organize today's presentation, and if I have any comments I will freely express them.

XIN ZHU　心　主

Elisabeth Rochat: The programme for today is the so-called heart governor, and I think we can begin with a study of some ideograms. At the last seminar in January we looked at the heart, *xin* (心), and we saw that the ideogram for heart is simply the form of a heart with the beginning of the aorta. In contrast to all the other viscera, there is no flesh radical in the composition of this ideogram. The only other exception is the triple heater, which we will see tomorrow.

The heart is essentially a void because the void is the only possible dwelling place for the spirits. Spirits can only rest and dwell in the void of the heart. The art of the heart, which is a famous discipline in Chinese philosophy, is the way to obtain and conserve this void which allows the spirits to be present and to impart spiritual essences and power to the blood. The blood is a body fluid, a red liquid which comes from the stomach and spleen, but the difference between this blood and other liquids in the body is that blood is infused with the power of the spirits of the heart.

The heart, as a void, has the possibility of receiving spiritual influences in the form of *shen* (神). There is also another ideogram *ling* (靈) which also means the reception of spiritual influences, and which is found in the names of the some of the points of the *shao yin* (少 陰) of the hand, the heart meridian. From all this emanates the radiance of the spirits, *shen ming* (神 明). This enables life to be led, but in a subtle way which is invisible and imperceptible. For this reason the names of the points on the heart meridian are not names like great this or greater that, but are just concerned with the spirits and with spiritual influx, and have names like small, very small, little and very little. This meridian ends at the smallest finger just in order to manifest this perceptible aspect of the void of the heart.

Now we come to see the other aspect of the heart, that which manifests its power on the middle finger, the longest and largest finger. The name is *xin zhu* (心 主). If you remember Su wen chapter 8 you will recall that the charge of the heart was to be the sovereign, *jun* (君), and master, *zhu* (主), and this *zhu* is the active aspect of this charge. The sovereign is a prince or a king, he who because of his lineage and ancestors and through his own virtue is the heart of a country or state, while the master is the one who is in charge of accomplishing things. The master has the necessary authority to complete the duties, be they governing a country or organizing a banquet.

The etymology of this character *zhu* (主) is found in Wieger lesson 83D: a lamp-stand with the flame rising. By extension, a man who spreads light, a lord, a master. [Wieger "Chinese Characters" published by Dover]. So, we have in this term master a more concrete and visible aspect, and you can see how the etymology of the ideogram is linked with the idea of fire. But you cannot push these associations too far!

This expression *xin zhu* (心 主) therefore means the heart in the function of master, not the heart as a void, but as master in charge of something. In charge of what? In charge of blood, *xue* (血), or in charge of the network of animation, *mai* (脈), carrying and transporting blood. The expressions *xin zhu xue* (心 主 血), the heart masters the blood, *xin zhu mai* (心 主 脈), the heart masters the network for animation perceptible at the pulses and *xin zhu xue mai* (心 主 血 脈), the heart masters the network for the circulation of blood, are very common in Chinese texts. So this is the more concrete, visible aspect of the power of the heart, and in this aspect you find the pathology. On the contrary, the void of the heart cannot have pathology. This expression *xin zhu*, heart master, always designates the meridian and the power and qualities of its particular *qi*. It never designates an organ or a viscera, only the function. The usual expression in Chinese to describe this meridian is the heart master of the hand, reflecting the power of the heart in activity, with the charge of mastering something.

Claude Larre: To consider something as a state of stillness, without any activity, and then to consider the same thing in the process of activity is the same thing as to speak of the way and the virtue, *dao de* (道 德). One distinction between the way and the virtue is that when you just contemplate what exists there is no image, there is just a stillness on your part awaiting a manifestation. To be awaiting a manifestation does not necessarily mean that something is manifest, you are just in the void. And that condition may lead you to the meaning of heart as just emptiness, for recollection or for the reception of something. But if that emptiness is real, even without any image from your mind, it may, by itself, be capable of operating something. When something exists, something may operate.

These two positions, the way and the virtue, the non-operation and the activity are so profound, so essential to the Chinese mind that it is quite natural that we would find them in this exposition on the two aspects of the heart. If the heart is the centre, if the heart is so important that you cannot even indicate what it is, then you understand that for mankind the heart is the seat of the way, it is nearly the same thing as the way. So if heart takes the place of the way, the virtue of the way has also to be expressed, and that would be by this other aspect of heart, heart mastering. But mastery is not mastery if there are no servants, so all the other organs come and make some kind of officialdom or a court for the sovereign. These remarks are very simple, but they have the intention of helping you understand that you are never able to speak of the heart as you are able to speak of the kidneys or liver, or any other *zang fu* (臟 府). The heart is elevated so high in our mind that we separate it, but the king is never so separate from the people and the officials that he is not in permanent relationship with them. He has his own privacy, but he is always in the mind of the people, and always in the mind of the officials.

So it is important to understand that the Chinese were more keen to observe how life functions than to observe parts of the anatomy, and if we really want to cure people we have to approach the functioning of life.

Elisabeth has reminded me of a certain part of the funeral rites. When they have disposed of the body and have prayed and made offerings for the three *hun* (魂), or the so-called soul, then something has to be done in the house where that person was master. They call a man from the village, usually a man of some authority, and inscribe the name of the deceased person on a tablet. The man of authority then places a red dot on it. This means that the tablet not only designates the deceased man, but has the power to make the memory of the man permanent in the house where he was once resident. When he was a living person he was acting as a visible authority, now he will be acting as an invisible authority.

Elisabeth Rochat: If you take this ideogram *zhu* (主) and add the fire radical on the left you have the meaning of a candle, *zhu* (炷). If you add the water radical you have an ideogram which means a flowing out or an outpouring of liquid, *zhu* (注).

Claude Larre: It means a normal and orderly flowing out from the vessel, not an overflowing.

Elisabeth Rochat: It is produced not through a loss of something but through a concentration of power: that is the flowing of a regular current producing in each place it passes a sort of concentration of power which allows all the required effects to be brought into being.

Claude Larre: The point is to make a difference between this and the *yuan* (原), source, which does not have so much usable power. It is necessary to have a source for the water, but this source, *yuan*, is more connected with the humidity of the ground.

One may say that the important thing is just the *zhu* itself. If you add the fire radical you have the idea that this candle is really giving light or warmth. If you add the water radical you have this place where the power of something (here it is water because of the radical) is collected.

Elisabeth Rochat: We can continue by adding the radical of wood to get the idea of a pillar, a support, perhaps for a house, or for the head on a body or for heaven and earth, *zhu* (柱). From all this we can see that in the expression *xin zhu* (心 主), heart master, there is an idea of movement, the movement of *qi*. *Xin zhu* is an activity, not something which remains static but something which is able to go everywhere with a great concentration of power, and to be like a master in every circumstance.

XIN BAO LUO 心 包 絡

Elisabeth Rochat: The other expression connected with this is *xin bao luo* (心 包 絡). *Xin* (心) is the heart. *Bao* (包) is like an envelope, like a matrix, because the etymology of this ideogram shows an embryo in the uterus. And the last ideogram, *luo* or *lo* (絡), is the same as is used in the so-called secondary pathways.

Question: Are these the secondary meridians, the *luo* meridians?

Elisabeth Rochat: Yes, but it is impossible to say secondary

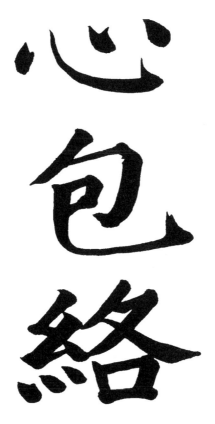

Xin bao luo

meridian. A meridian is either a main meridian or it is not a meridian.

Claude Larre: This is a very important point. The expressions generally used in books are 'secondary meridian' or 'primary meridian'. A meridian is really a sign that heaven is, in one way or another, giving its authority in order that such things could exist. The will of heaven is not seen in itself, it has to be received by the earthly aspect of life, and the combination of the reception by earth and the communication of this power from heaven is what makes life exist. So when you look at the face of a person, you see some sort of earthly expression, but at the same time on the face itself you see the expression of life. This can give you so much inspiration that you see that heaven has been manifesting through earth. It is impossible to separate what heaven and earth are doing, but through what exists you are able to make a distinction between them since you are made of them.

Elisabeth Rochat: Bao (包) has this idea of enveloping or enclosing something very precious. It is to surround or to envelop, but also to protect and to maintain. Everything is brought together in order to maintain it, in just the same way that a woman carries a foetus or a bird broods on its eggs. It is the idea of enveloping something that is very vital, and perhaps also gathering, surrounding, bringing together all that is different or diverse to hold it in some kind of unity. If you add the radical for flesh to this ideogram *bao* (胞) then you have the idea of a matrix, and everything that resembles a matrix.

Question: The uterus?

Claude Larre: The problem is that we do not know whether the uterus has as many accepted usages in English to encompass not only the materiality of it but also all its functions.

Comment: Matrix is a very good word.

Elisabeth Rochat: And a particular example of this matrix can be the womb or the uterus.

Claude Larre: Uterus would be much too restricted.

Elisabeth Rochat: It's not just a womb, but the concept of the womb. It's amusing that if we add the ideogram for building, it becomes cooking, the cook, or the place where the meals are prepared. It is the place where something is prepared.

Claude Larre: Carefully prepared!

Elisabeth Rochat : *Luo* (絡) has the thread of silk radical on the left, and the part on the right means to go on its own way. When you go your own way in the manner of a silk thread you have the impression of weaving fibres, not quite separate threads, but like cotton wool made of silk. Or to make another analogy, between the fruit of an orange and the skin there is the white pulp or pith, and this is like the *luo*. Therefore, it is a whole network of filaments which intertwine, envelop and serve as an intermediary, wrapping or encircling something. But this is not done in the same manner as an envelope, it is rather a multiplication or an increasing of the possible relations, links and connections which attach one thing to another, just as the white pith in the orange links the fruit inside to the skin outside.

What we call the *luo*, the secondary pathways of energy, are just everything in the body which make up the multiplicity of filaments which reach up to our outer skin. When a meridian takes a *luo* relationship with its coupled organ, for example the lung meridian with the large intestine, it is just that the *qi* of the lung meridian is encircling, with multiple relationships, the power of the large intestine. In *luo* there is this idea of the penetration and occupation of a space, and of course there are *luo* everywhere in the body.

So what does the expression *bao luo* (包 絡) mean when it is linked specifically to the heart? It means that the heart, which is presented as a void, needs not only a protection, an enveloping of this void, but also a permanent connection, a network for relationships.

Claude Larre: The void is something solid, firm, and important, nearly visible, but invisible.

Elisabeth Rochat: A sovereign or president of a republic who embodies his function well is like a void.

Claude Larre: That can be seen very well in the state of political affairs in France. If the prime minister is able to do his work when the president of the republic has all the power, the only way that can be possible is for the president to create a void so that there is room enough for the prime minister to operate through the government. The point is that the prime minister should not let people think that the president of the republic is of no importance. If he is able to give the impression that the president is very, very important, so important that he has nothing to do, then he has succeeded. The same thing goes for the queen and her government in England. But the competition between the queen, or king, and the government has a long tradition here, so it runs more easily, as it is supposed to! Maybe that was the situation with Disraeli and Victoria, when Disraeli was in fact doing everything but always referring to Queen Victoria as if she was the most important. This gives you the interplay of the two aspects: the immense void is so important that it does nothing. But if there is no void there is no room for the prime minister to operate.

Elisabeth Rochat: The void of the heart can only manifest

through the radiance of the spirits, but looking at the other side we see the manifestion of the heart in the form of this envelope. What we call the envelope of the heart can perhaps also be seen as all the membranes around the heart, and there are ancient texts in the classics which say that this is so. Then we can go further and say that it is the pericardium, or not just the pericardium but the myocardium. If the heart of the heart shelters the spirits then the invisible aspects of the heart must be enveloped and protected, but they must also be manifested in a visible aspect. That is to say Buckingham Palace is not the queen, but it gives a good impression of the royalty in England. It represents the crown. This is linked to the idea of emperor. So I think these envelopes are to be taken as everything that manifests the visible aspects of the heart.

Claude Larre: Everything Elisabeth has been saying about the envelopes of the heart can only be said if we call the heart this kind of internal void, this median void. Most of the time in the classical texts what will be called the heart will be a more manifest and more active kind of heart, and it is because of this that the expression *xin bao luo* is not found in the Su wen, and is only found two or three times in the Ling shu. They talk only of the heart, and we know that the heart can represent these two aspects of void and activity, but in the classical language the context itself is sufficient to determine which aspect they are talking about.

The expression *xin bao luo* designates the two aspects necessary to a central power: the guard and protection with the idea of an envelope which encircles and prepares for life, and then all the communication systems without which no authority can exist. For example, if in time of war there are no messengers, or if the sovereign does not know what is happening, then there is disorder. In the pathology of the heart, which covers the pathology of the heart as a communicator or in its enveloping aspect, there are a lot of disorders and illnesses which are the result of losing contact with the spirits that are in the heart. A good example of this breakdown in communication is seen in the case of *tan* (痰), phlegm, when this obstructs or veils the orifices of the heart with resulting physical and mental symptoms.

I would like to come back for one moment to try to pull together all that has been said about the heart of man. If we understand that heaven is necessarily the first expression of the void then we see that earth is ready for form. It is impossible to create form other than from the void, and the void has no meaning if there is no form to be changed in the void. The highest combination of heaven and earth is given in the meeting which we call man.

Man must maintain this void in order to relate to heaven, and must be receptive to any sort of force coming from heaven and reflected in the void in order to change and develop. The development of man is seen in the centre of the body, which is the heart. It is very difficult to keep the same void which we have in heaven in the heart, but if we can, then the spirits will come. The only way to have communication with heaven is to be so void in the heart that the spirits, *shen* (神), can come and go. Then heaven / heart is understood as this master who is not doing, who is very active but active in non-interferring. That is the reason why in Lao zi it is said that the sage has no heart himself, he simply takes the heart of the people for his own heart. The necessity for the emptiness of the void is seen here.

But in contrast with this role or function of mastery, *zhu* (主), we have the co-functions of the *bao* (包), the enclosing aspect and the *luo* (絡), the connective aspect. Here again it is necessary that something of the void is kept, and this is done by means of the envelope. The envelope has the function of protecting the void, but if you are too greatly protected there is no longer a relationship with the outside, and you cannot exert any influence. So from this void and from this envelope it is necessary that there are emissaries and messengers, the *luo*.

The main point is to keep in mind the fact that the difficulty we have is not with the ideas but with the language. The language, English or French or whatever, makes things appear with their forms, but what we need is not only to see the forms but to see the void which is receiving the forms. The continued presence of the void is necessary, and it is only with that concept that the regulation of heaven, earth and man can be seen in every particular detail of our life.

Elisabeth Rochat: There is a text from Zhuang zi chapter 2 which talks about the life of the universe which can be applied to the heart:

> *Suppose that there is a true master, one sees no indication of his existence. You see his actions but without seeing his visible form. Thus, for example, a body is composed of a hundred bones, of nine orifices and of six viscera. Of all these components which one should I like? Do you like them all? Do you prefer certain ones? Are they all servants? Are these servants incapable of ruling themselves? Must they each in turn become master and servant? If there is a true prince, our knowledge and our ignorance about him neither increases nor diminishes in any way his truth.*

This is reality and we can apply this text to the heart. The form of the heart as prince and sovereign is not perceptible, while the activity and authority in which it takes form becomes perceptible. Its servants are innumerable. They are all these envelopes and connections: the *tan zhong* (膻 中), sea of *qi* in the chest, all the organs and all the network of animation, *mai* (脈), each having some kind of mastery in their sphere.

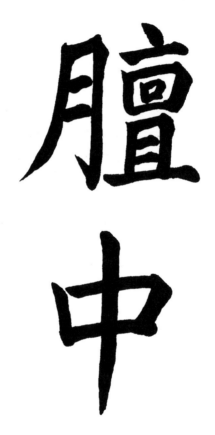

Tan zhong

NEI JING TEXTS

SU WEN CHAPTER 8

Elisabeth Rochat: Now we are going to look at texts drawn from the Nei jing to clarify this other aspect of the heart. We can begin with Su wen chapter 8, The Secret Treatise of the Spiritual Orchid. In this chapter Qi Bo gives a definition of each of the twelve charges of the twelve viscera. But there is no mention of *xin bao luo* (心 包 絡), or *xin zhu* (心 主). Instead we find *tan zhong* (膻 中), the sea of *qi.* As I said before, *xin bao luo* is an expression which does not appear in the Su wen. Chapter 8 says:

> *Tan zhong has the charge of resident as well as envoy, chen shi* (臣 使).

Envoy of whom? Of the heart, the master. So in the charge of *tan zhong* we can refine this concept of a whole crowd of messengers, ambassadors and servants and see that it is in fact *tan zhong* that effectively takes charge of the organs in each particular situation and brings the orders and the light of the spirits of the heart. Thus Su wen chapter 8 is saying that for all the *qi* in the body the point of departure for propagation throughout the whole organism is the sea of *qi* in the chest. This, of course, does not prevent the lungs from being a master of *qi* in so far as they give the rhythm that makes life.

Question: Where has all this *qi* suddenly appeared from?

Elisabeth Rochat: The *qi* is concentrated at *tan zhong* which is the sea of *qi*. The definition of *tan zhong* is in Ling shu chapter 33, and refers to the *qi* of the whole organism.

Question: I don't understand the connection between this whole army of messengers to the heart and the text.

Elisabeth Rochat: You have to refer to this text of Su wen chapter 8. The first charge was that of the heart, which is the sovereign and master. For this reason all ministers, servants or envoys are ministers, servants or envoys from the sovereign. You cannot be the minister for a minister.

Question: So *chen* (臣) means servant?

Elisabeth Rochat: Any kind of servant or minister is a servant of the king. And *shi* (使) is an envoy, a person who has been delegated to do something or send a message or an order which has come from a superior. In the hierarchy of Su wen chapter 8 before *tan zhong* (膻 中) we only have the heart which has the charge of sovereign and master, and afterwards we have the lungs with the charge of minister and chancellor, and then the liver and gallbladder. The linking of the charge of servant and envoy with the previous charge of sovereign and lord is found in Chinese commentaries, for example in the 17th century there is this commentary:

> *Tan zhong is located in the middle of the thorax between the two breasts.*

We can just comment here that *ming men* (命 門) is also in a space between the two kidneys, and this is a parallel with the spreading out of light from the heart and this accumulation of *qi* between the two breasts. The text continues:

> *Tan zhong is the sea of qi. The heart commands [xin zhu] and it is the lord, and there must be a sending out of the orders, messages and decrees. Tan zhong governs and commands qi to spread out and to distribute the yin as well as the yang.*

That is all the different kinds of *qi*, the nutritive as well as the defensive, that in the *yin* meridians as well as in the *yang* meridians. So this text, which is an ancient commentary, puts all the *yin yang* propagation of *qi* in a postition of dependence on the charge of the sovereign and master, and links that to the propagation of decrees and orders.

Claude Larre: When we start with this power at the highest level, and we say that the charge there is to be sovereign and master, what we finally get is the radiance of the spirits, something proper to the heart, and nearly invisible, but seen in the *shen ming* (神 明). The result is a person's joy. There are two kinds of joy, an excited joy, *xi* (喜), and a more profound joy, *le* (樂). Joy is more visible than the *shen ming,* that radiance of the spirits, therefore we can understand that *tan zhong* is something more visible than *xin* (心). The heart is so void, and *tan zhong* is so expressive, but that does not exactly mean that the location is really physical. As far as I understand it, when we are talking of heart we know that we should not take it too physically. We go through the location to understand where life is operating, it is a door to get to somewhere where life is more manageable.

Elisabeth Rochat: What is a sea of *qi?* It is a function which receives the full power of the *qi* and circulates it throughout the body. The specific charge of *tan zhong* is the rapport and connection with the heart, because it is through this *qi,* whose rhythm is ensured by the lungs, that the orders of the heart are passed on, just as the spirits of the heart invisibly impregnate the blood. The *qi,* being omnipresent in the body, is a factotem for the heart. It is present wherever any kind of exchange takes place, full of the direction of life given by the heart. Perhaps it is because of this power of the heart and the upper heater that the *qi* can find a unity and fidelity to the true being.

This can be seen, for example, in *zong qi* (宗 氣), ancestral *qi*, which only exists at the level of *tan zhong*. This is also the *qi* that makes the heart beat. *Zong qi* gives the idea of some kind of convergence, and it also has the sense of being a way in which *qi* is able to exist with all its different functions at all levels of the being. This will be seen again when we come to the triple heater.

Another aspect of all this is that the heart has mastery over the *mai* (脈) which are all the pathways of animation and circulation, of the *qi* as well as the blood. So it is interesting to see that the void of the heart, which subtly allows all these circulations, reveals its visible side through the mastery that it has over all the pathways of animation in the body. This applies to all that we call transformation. The commentaries repeat that it is the void of the heart that allows transformation, and it is through the *qi* that transformation can take place within the body.

It is interesting to see that *qi* and blood are each linked in their different way to the power of the heart, helped at the same time by the auxillary power of the lungs which give the instinctive rhythm for life. If the laws are good and well adapted to the people, and are well distributed everywhere, the people will be happy and there will be elation and joy! That is the same thing as saying that if the blood and the *qi* circulate everywhere in the body, nourishing, defending and transforming, being where they are needed in such a way as to make you feel very good in yourself, you can experience this feeling of joy which is characteristic of being alive.

Claude Larre: At this point something has to be said about treatment. Usually people come and ask to be treated in order to be given back this feeling of elation and joy. And if after the treatment they do feel well disposed it is because harmonization and regularity have been obtained through the hands and mind of the practitioner. But this is only at the level of number five. If the treatment is done quickly, without any profundity, after a time the feeling of excitement and joy will disappear, and the patient will come back in order to get another treatment to restore it. You will have a permanent patient because your effect is not going higher than number five. But if through your treatment you are really able to set the heart in its own place with the result that the *shen ming* are radiant, then the consequence will be that numbers two, three, four and five are all regulated and will be so for a much more extended time because your treatment has been at the level of number one. So the sort of treatment that can be given depends upon the practitioner, his or her personal identity, morality and ability to go higher. I am sure that some of what the texts call 'great acupuncturists' will always get to this first place from which everything flows, but those who are good but not excellent will not reach that level, even if the patient is pleased for a month!

Question:. Su wen chapter 8 describes the heart as being lord and master. Is the master side what you were first talking about as *xin zhu?*

Claude Larre: You cannot divide it into one or the other. When it is stated in Su wen chapter 8, you may as easily say it is *xin* (心), heart, as *zhu* (主), master. If you take out *zhu* you say of course the heart is the lord, but the lord is doing his mastering, and you reconstruct from the text something which is *zhu.* The heart really does have the role of the master, but this is an explanation which is true in your mind but which is not the proper Chinese text. The danger comes when you want to take something which is true but is not the wording of the text, and transfer it to another text. The connection between the understanding of a notion and the way the Chinese are expressing it through characters is so close that you are not supposed to make any separation inside the text. The more we know the texts only through the English translation the more impossible it becomes.

Elisabeth Rochat: To be sovereign and master is the invisible aspect of the function of the heart, and the radiance of the spirits stems from it. The radiance of the spirits is intangible, but elation and joy are more tangible and these, along with such things as blood and *mai* are the manifestations of the power of the heart. This is the other side of the heart. In Su wen chapter 8 after the presentation of the 12 charges there is this sentence:

> *If the master radiates (virtue) those under him will be at peace. Through this the nurturing of life will yield longevity.*

Peace is an indication that everything is functioning as well as it can with no disturbance. On the other hand, if the master does not radiate virtue the 12 charges will be in danger, causing a closing and blocking of communication which will injure the body. It is essential that good communication is ensured at every level, and it is absolutely vital that this is so at the central level of life, in the heart.

So the meaning of *xin zhu* is found in all the communications, attachments and connections by which the heart radiates the light of the spirits. This permits the blood to be blood and the *qi* to be *qi*. It allows all the pathways of animation to not only be pathways for the blood and *qi* but also to be the intermediaries through which all the commandments and orders of the sovereign are passed and distributed.

LING SHU CHAPTER 35

Elisabeth Rochat: Now we'll look at a text from Ling shu chapter 35 which gives a close textual relationship between *tan zhong* and *xin zhu:*

Tan zhong is the imperial palace, jin cheng (禁 城), *of xin zhu.*

The text makes a very close connection between the heart spreading its activity and the sea of *qi* in the chest. The sea of *qi* is the heart's servant and messenger but also its protector. So you can see that *tan zhong* and *xin bao luo* are interlinked, and are actually just different ways of seeing the same reality, given different expression through the centuries. In some periods they talk more of *xin bao luo*, and in others not, and the Chinese today even have the same difficulties as we do in understanding.

LING SHU CHAPTER 71

Huang Di asked: The mai of the shao yin of the hand, alone, has no yu (俞). *Why?*

Qi Bo replied: The shao yin of the hand is the mai of the heart. The heart is the grand master, da zhu (大 主), *of the five zang and six fu, the residence of the essences/spirits, jing shen* (精 神). *When this zang is solid and firm, the perverse influences cannot be admitted. If they are admitted then the heart is injured and if the heart is injured, the spirits, shen* (神), *leave and if the shen leave it is death. For this reason, when the perverse*

*influences are in the heart, they are in the enveloping
network, bao luo* (包 絡). *The bao luo is the mai of xin
zhu* (心 主). *This is why it alone has no yu* (俞).

*Huang di said: The shao yin, alone, not having a yu, is
it then never ill?*

*Qi Bo said: Its meridian on the exterior is ill, but the zang
is not ill. This is why the meridian is taken (needled)
only at the end of the pointed bone that is located behind
the palm of the hand (ie shen men* 神 門, *Ht 7).*

Elisabeth Rochat: What is the meaning of this *yu* (俞)? It is
not exactly a point in the way that the ideogram *xue* (穴) is
translated as point. *Xue* is a cave, an hollow, a grotto, an
underground place from which something springs up, or
from which you can make something spring up, and it is
the most usual term for designating a point. But there are
other ideograms which are also translated as point, and
this *yu* is one of them.

Yu is usually written with the flesh radical on the left side,
(腧), but it can equally be found with the radical for vehicle.
In that case it is pronounced *shu* (輸), and that explains
why the back *yu* points are also referred to as *shu* points.
When you have the vehicle radical it adds the idea of
transportation and action at a distance, with the term *yu*
there is the idea of a place where there is the presence of a

vital injection, a transfer.

Claude Larre: The Wieger reference for this character is lesson 14F: a junction of a few planks, forming a boat to go up the river. It says up the river not along the river and this is important. What it means is that there are places where if a puncture is made for this sort of treatment, then the flux of life is so well organized that there will be an effect upwards. A reconciliation of the disorder is obtained through the puncturing of the placc where the vital flux is so well organized that it goes back to the origin. The river is similar to the flux of life, but why the boat? Because if you have to go up the river it is better to embark in a boat!

Elisabeth Rochat: We use this character *xue* (穴) in an almost neutral capacity. You can say that the heart meridian has nine points, and this would be *xue* because it implies nothing, neither a treatment nor the absence of treatment, it just implies the places where there is an underground reserve, or there are stages for the progression of life when it is formed. The other terms *yu* (俞) and *shu* (輸) are used when it is a question of an effect being produced, or an effect that needs to be produced, as for example in groups of well-defined points such as the *yu* or *shu* points of the back or the points that are between the fingers and elbows which are represented by the points of the five elements.

In this text when it says that the *shao yin* of the hand has no *yu* it does not mean that there are no points on the heart meridian, it just means that the effects are not comparable with other meridians. If the heart is nothing other than this central void, or this profound unity in the being which is the residence of the spirits, it cannot be linked to a particular season, and hardly to a particular element, so it is not possible to try and regulate it in relationship to elements and seasons or to *qi* and blood. This is why it says here that the heart meridian has no *yu*. The ancient texts still attribute the points on the heart meridian to the different elements, but it is also true that the points on the heart meridian are very rarely used in this particular way in relationship to the five elements.

Claude Larre: I shall add a very short story. On my way back to Paris from China 20 years ago I stopped in Rome and visited the general of the Jesuits. I thought it was a good opportunity to ask for a certain personal favour, and I tried to formulate something. But he said, 'Stop there, I give you all the permission you need.' In fact I had no special permission because he was ready to give permission for everything, thus sending me back to a more ordinary superior who would ask me specific reasons for my requests. Since the heart is the sovereign he is not supposed to give a special effect, he is there as reference for all the *zang* and all the body. It is not that he is not co-operating, but that he is co-operating with so many others that in taking charge of the whole he cannot take charge of the detail.

Elisabeth Rochat: For this reason the *mai* of *shao yin* of the hand (the heart meridian) has no *yu*, and if you look at Ling shu chapter 2 or other texts such as the Nan jing, when they talk of the *yu* points or the points of the so-called five elements on the heart meridian, you always have the names of the points of the *xin zhu*, heart master, meridian. For example in Ling shu chapter 2 it says that the *mai* of the heart comes out at *zhong chong* (中 衝) which is the name of point nine of the *xin zhu* meridian. In this case it gives the exact location of the point so wc know that they are talking about the *xin zhu* meridian.

The Ling shu also cites the five points of the *xin zhu* pathway up to the *he* (合) point at the elbow, and then it says that this is the *shao yin* of the hand. So there was certainly some hesitation in ancient times between calling it the *shao yin* or the *xin zhu*. There were even some schools which only had 11 meridians. For example in the Mawangdui tomb dating from about 162 BC, medical texts were found which listed the meridians as only 11 and the missing one was either the heart, *shao yin,* or the heart master, *xin zhu* meridian. It is difficult to know exactly which because the names are a bit mixed up.

What is important is to see the heart expressed in a central pathway down the hand, and also that the heart is in some way inexpressible. In the era just after Christ, it is difficult to be exact, the 12 meridians were categorized and became more definite. But it does seem that the points of the *shao yin* are not used in the same way as others, and this text of Ling shu chapter 71 explains that this is because the *shao yin* of the hand expresses the heart as the grand master of the five *zang* and the six *fu*, and as such cannot relate with them at the same level. The heart is at the upper level, the dwelling of the *jing shen*, the highest level of vitality of life, the interpenetration of essences by the spirits.

Classic commentators on this section of the Ling shu say that the lord and master resides in non-action, and the *bao luo*, the enveloping network of the heart, are the delegates of the heart, making all the *qi* and blood circulate, communicating and carrying out orders. So while the *jing shen*, esences/spirits, or vital spirit, are stored in the heart, everything that emanates from them circulates in activity which is expressed by this other meridian, *xin zhu*. And it is on this other meridian that you find the places to regulate all that comes from the execution of the heart's orders. The heart within the heart, the void that shelters the spirits, cannot be subjected to perverse influences. The spirits are unalterable, unchangeable, either they are present or they are not.

Claude Larre: It is something like the light of the sun, you cannot destroy it, but you can cover it. And when we say there is no light, it is not that there is no light, but that there is no way for the light to shine through.

J. R. Worsley maintains that you should consider the patient as how he would be if he were healthy in order that your treatment reaches the authenticity of the individual. The patient you have before you is not really the person who exists, he is more or less covered by certain obstacles which you are supposed to remove. The reason for this is that the *shen* (神) and the heart are made for one another, and if the *shen* are no longer there it might be that the essences are not there, and if the essences are not there maybe the *qi* is not there. But if we call back the *qi* the health of the patient will be restored, the spirits will return and radiate again.

Elisabeth Rochat: So finally, the heart itself cannot be ill, but all its ways of expression and communication can be ill or disordered. This is to say that it is only the power of the heart that can be regulated. The deep direction of life is not regulated through the *qi* and the blood, but is regulated in the way that the sun regulates life on Earth, and can be touched on the meridian of the heart, and in particular by the point which is the door of the spirits, *shen men* (神 門).

NAN JING TEXTS

NAN JING DIFFICULTY 25

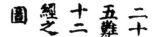

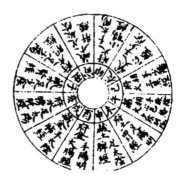

*There are 12 meridians. Five zang and six fu, that makes
11. This additional meridian, what sort of meridian is it?*

*As to this meridian, the shao yin of the hand and the xin
zhu are separate mai. The xin zhu and the three heaters
are related internally/externally. These have a name but
do not have a form. It is because of this that one speaks
of the meridians in saying that there are 12.*

Elisabeth Rochat: The first part of this difficulty 25 means that each of the five *zang* and six *fu* have a meridian, *mai* (脈), but the heart has a double *mai* to express this duality or two-sidedness of its nature. Here it says that *xin zhu,* heart master, and the three heaters are related *biao/li,* internally/externally, and *xin zhu* is not to be taken as a different *zang* from the heart, but just as an aspect of the heart in activity.

Another link between the heart and the three heaters is that they both have a name but do not have a form. *Xin zhu* is the name given only to the *qi* in the meridian, it never means the organ. So, when in the Nan jing they ask why there are 12 meridians, the answer is because the heart has two linked to itself.

NAN JING DIFFICULTY 39

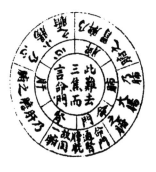

The classics say that the fu are five and that the zang are six. How is this?

Six fu, yes; but there are really only five fu. Five zang, but there can also be six zang. This is because one speaks of the kidneys as having a double storage, liang cang (兩 藏): *on the left is the kidney and on the right is ming men* (命 門). *Ming men is the place where the essences spirits, jing/shen* (精 神), *live; where man stores the essences (sperm) and woman connects the reproductive organs. Its qi is in free communication with the kidneys. It is because of this that one says that the zang are six. But how can the fu be five? The five zang each have a fu; the three heaters are indeed a fu, but they do not depend on any of the five zang. It is because of this that it is said that the fu are five.*

Elisabeth Rochat: At first it seems that there is contradiction, but in fact it is because we are not looking from the same perspective. In difficulty 25 we were talking about the 12 meridians, and within that perspective the reply was made of a double expression of *qi* for the heart, *shao yin* and *xin zhu,* and within this expression *xin zhu* is in a *biao/li* relationship with the three heater. But in this difficulty 39 the question relates to the *zang* and *fu* themselves, and the reply is the same as it is in other places in the Nan jing and the Nei jing, that when we speak of the six *zang* the *xin bao luo* is never included as one of the six, it is always the kidneys which are seen as having a double action. The heart is for the expression of life from a central void, and the kidneys are for the keeping and conserving of the deepest foundation of life, and the origin of life itself which is *ming men.* So when you speak of six *zang* there will always be the five *zang* plus this primitive storage which is the other aspect of the kidneys.

This is clarified in other texts of the Ling shu, for example chapters 2 and 47. In Ling shu chapter 47 the kidneys are linked to the triple heater and to the bladder. This means that when we speak of the *zang* and the *fu* it is the kidneys

that are double, and when we talk of the expression of the
qi of the mai, or the meridians, it is the heart which is
double. We will see this again with the triple heater.

We may just mention that there is a vital enveloping of the
heart as for the kidneys. For the heart it is the protective
envelope, bao (包), around its void and spiritual power. For
the kidneys it is the protective envelope, bao, of the germ of
life, of the flowing source for the development of my own
life, or, in the case of the pregnant woman, of another
embryonic life.

Question: Can you say more about *ming men?*

Elisabeth Rochat: Ming men (命 門) is the original, anterior,
primitive aspect, and it cannot be expressed by itself. If
there is a *ming men* there is a beginning of life, of a particular
life, and afterwards this fire of life can become the foundation
for the power of the heart. In the body of an adult it becomes
like a minister, the ministerial fire at the service of the
heart. This is because as an adult the person is in full
possession of himself, his spirits are in charge and manifest,
but only if he conforms at each instant with each part of
his being to his own original essence which is first manifest
as *ming men.* As the human being matures the spirits are
the expression of the original expression of *ming men. Ming*
(命) is destiny, and destiny in the Chinese sense of the
term, is the way in which one's life unfolds, conforming

with what we have received from heaven. That is, conformity with one's own nature in order to become what one is. Destiny is an unfolding of original nature. *Men* (門) is the gate or door.

Claude Larre: There is a simpler way to explain this: a door is a door, and a room is a room. The door is opening into the room, and the room is the heart. The room has to be empty, and if it is empty the spirits will stay inside. *Ming men* is the door, and the spirits will always come through the door, and will always be stored in that same room.

Question: Can you explain how that transition is made in children?

Claude Larre: Well, when we are talking of children we have a room in the making and a door in the making, but the door is made before the room. It is always easier to make an opening and then to organize it! *Ming men* is some sort of first condition of the embryo and the slow formation of all the parts which go to make the human being. The heart is beginning in the mother, and as far as the embryo is concerned, some sort of separation is made between the heart of the mother and the heart of the child. But we know that the link between the mother and child can never really be cut because it was there at the beginning, and what has been there at the beginning must stay to the end, even if it has to change. This is very clear if we understand that when we talk of heart we are not referring to this piece of flesh in the chest, but to the organization of life. It is certain that at the early stages of the embryo all the responsibility for life is on the mother, but through its formation the embryo aquires more responsibility and the *du mai* (督 脈), *ren mai* (任 脈) and *chong mai* (衝 脈) rely on each other in order to transform the newly-born into an adult. But in as much as separation occurs, it occurs with some sort of subordination because the mother is always referring to the child and the child is always referring to the mother. This is quoted in Lao zi when it says:

> *When I see the child I think of the mother and when I am with the mother I am thinking of the child.*

Question: So the independence of the child is when he or she starts to bring his own *ming men* into his heart.

Claude Larre: You may say that. The independence, the *ming men* is your fate, but your fate is integrated within the fate of the lineage, and that's the reason why there is the cult of ancestors. That is the Chinese concept of life: the individual life is to be referred to the life of the ancestors. One is free and dependent at the same time. This is quite the opposite of the more usual Western concept that the more dependent you are the less free you are. Of course if the person you are dependent on does not have the same concept as you then it will not be easy!

Question: Is that maturation process the same process that is also mentioned in some texts about transformation of *jing* (精) into *shen* (神)?

Elisabeth Rochat: There is no transformation of *jing* into *shen.* Essences, *jing* (精), are just the means by which spirits express themselves, and essences can be *qi* and blood and so on. But spirits are spirits, and untransformable. We cannot transform our spirits in any way, we are just able to keep them or let them go, to allow them to express the heavenly way in us or not.

Claude Larre: The difficulty comes from the difference of vocabulary between Chinese words and English words. When we call on the spirits in Chinese we know that they are pertaining to heaven, but when we talk of spirits in English or French we pretend that they are so close to our own mind that we may influence them and make them conform more or less to our wishes, which is not true.

Question: But some meditations did attempt to transform *jing* and *qi* into *shen* ?

Claude Larre: I am sure this process of working depends on whether people have been able to make a good translation, since when the Chinese say 'transformed' they mean that what you have been seeing one way you now need to be able to see another way. This does not mean it has changed.

TRIPLE HEATER

san jiao

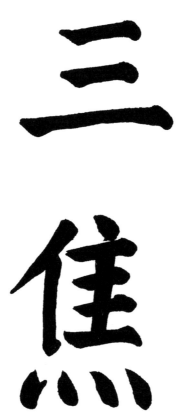

San jiao

THE TRIPLE HEATER

SAN JIAO 三 焦

THE IDEOGRAM SAN 三

Elisabeth Rochat: In this expression triple heater, *san jiao* (三 焦), the ideogram *jiao* is important of course, but the ideogram *san,* three or triple is also very important because three is the number of all that is held between the two poles. One is for the unity, and then you have a separation which gives two. This is *yin* and *yang* and heaven and earth. But between these two, in our living world, you have a perpetual exchange of influx, and for this reason you add another stroke to two and you have three. This graphically indicates all the exchange which takes place in the median space.

Three is the number of mankind because mankind, being between heaven and earth, best represents the influx of heaven and earth in a perpetual exchange and compenetration. For this reason three is also the special number of *qi*, because everything which is exchanged between the two poles of the median space is *qi*. All exchanges, all transformations of life, take place here at the level of three.

THE IDEOGRAM JIAO 焦

Elisabeth Rochat: At the bottom of this ideogram is the fire radical. You can write this radical in two ways, like flames rising up (which is used at the side of an ideogram) or as it is here like little flames under a kettle. These are the small flames that make pots simmer, like simmering a number of ingredients in water to make a delicious soup. You have to be French to understand the triple heater!

The upper part of the ideogram is a bird without a tail. According to Wieger lesson 126A the etymology of this ideogram is a bird being submitted to the action of fire, a fried or roast chicken perhaps. But this is not enough of an explanation, because what is the meaning of this lack of tail feathers? The bird is clearly not meant for flight, but everything else is well linked together, and in good relationship. Following from this idea, if you add the radical for vegetation to the top of the ideogram you have a character meaning bananas (蕉). Why? Because when bananas are on the tree they are all linked together in a tight bunch. If you add the silk thread radical you have another ideogram, *wei* (維), with the meaning of a lot of filaments which you can find in vegetables or textiles. If you add the water radical you have the idea of anchoring a boat, the link by which the boat is connected to the earth or to land. So you can see that these ideograms are all related to the idea of an attachment or joining, a connection or a cord which is the main cord in a net. Symbolically it is what gives the fundamental structure of life in society, in order to maintain and keep this kind of life well. Interestingly the character *wei* is the same one as in the *yin* or *yang wei mai* of the eight extraordinary meridians.

The meaning of *jiao* is that all the elements of the body are well linked together and converge on the same stem, which can also be seen in the feathers of a bird or bananas on a tree. At the same time there is this kind of fire which provides the necessary warmth to be alive and to transform *qi* and so on. If you substitute the radical for illness you have an ideogram with the meaning of being very thin and emaciated, lacking strength, and diminishing through suffering or pain. This is not just a medical term, but a common one for a state of complete exhaustion of the being.

NEI JING TEXTS

SU WEN CHAPTER 4

Elisabeth Rochat: Now that you have a general idea of what the three heaters are we can immediately have a look at the Nei jing and see first in the Su wen what information we have about the triple heater.

Su wen chapter 4 presents the five *zang* and six *fu* . The five *zang* are liver, heart, spleen, lung and kidneys and they are all *yin.* The six *fu* are gallbladder, stomach, large intestine, small intestine, bladder and triple heater and they are all *yang.* The only commentary I will make on that is that we have a presentation of the five *zang* and six *fu* and that the triple heater is always one of the six *fu.* It is not like the *xin zhu* or *xin bao luo* which is never a *zang* because it is just an aspect of the heart.

There are five *zang* because five is the number of the compenetration of the various qualities of *qi* on the earth and under heaven which are necessary to prepare and develop the knot of life. But six is another thing. Six is the number of the maintenance of this life through all the circulation and animation of *qi*. There are five elements on the Earth, but there are six types of *qi* or climates, for example cold, heat or wind. And this is something that is often repeated in the commentaries on the Nei jing and Nan jing, that the *zang* work more on the model of the five elements, while the *fu* work more on the model of the six *qi* and six climates. Of course there is also compenetration, and the joining of the two which allows all the transformations which are life.

SU WEN CHAPTER 11

Elisabeth Rochat: There is another presentation of the *fu* in Su wen chapter 11. The stomach, large intestine, small intestine, triple heater and bladder are named. These five *fu* are produced by the *qi* of heaven, and the *qi* is in the image of heaven and thus diffuses, but does not keep or store. So when you have five *fu* represented in the digestive tract it is not the triple heater that is absent but the gallbladder. The triple heater has all these aspects of reception, transformation, diffusion and elimination, even at the level of digestion. This is what is meant when it is said in the Neijing Jingyi that the three heaters are 'the pathways for the entry and exit of liquids and cereals'. This refers not only to the act of swallowing and excreting, but to everything that allows me to receive and introduce something into my body that is other than myself, something that comes from outside. It is also that which gives the ability to eliminate everything that cannot be integrated and assimilated into my being.

Between these two activities are all the transformations governed by the triple heater. The triple heater gives the unity to all these operations between entry and exit. The details may be governed by one organ or another, but the whole thing is governed by the triple heater, so it gives a unity to all this functioning. Between entry and exit there is all the transmission, all the circulation, all the transformation and this is also the best definition of the *fu* of the digestive tract, as is said in Su wen chapter 11. The triple heater is therefore the *fu* par excellence since it encompasses all the possible transformations of *qi*, and is the greatest agent for circulation. It is indeed a *fu* which retains and stores nothing, but which makes everything circulate in various ways to distribute *qi* throughout the body, and through the *qi* ensures the circulation of liquids in the body right up until their evacuation.

We will see, particularly in the Ling shu, that the triple heater is rooted at the deepest level of being. The Nan jing tells us that the triple heater has a very close relationship with *ming men*, that it develops throughout the whole body and that its influence extends right up to the outer layers of the skin. We will also see that it represents the mixing of water and fire, allowing the development of all life.

SU WEN CHAPTER 8

The triple heater is responsible for the opening up of passages and irrigation. The waterways stem from it.

Elisabeth Rochat: If we look at Su wen chapter 8, the first thing we see is that the triple heater can break through passages and pathways. It has the concentrated strength of *shao yang* (少 陽) which allows passing through obstacles and a clearing of the ways so that all the irrigation and streams in the body can circulate freely and keep the *qi* moving.

The character for irrigation, *du* (瀆), is a picture of a small channel of irrigation in a field, and it is the same as you find in one of the points on the triple heater meridian, *si du* (四瀆), TH 9. This ideogram *du* shows how you can make a piece of ground fertile by hollowing out the earth and making a pathway for circulation between the river and the field. It is the whole network of these small canals or channels which comprise the whole system of irrigation, drainage and evacuation. For example, in a town this would be the drainage and sewage system. All this would be represented by the ideogram *du* (瀆).

It is obvious that the most important thing is to ensure free communication. There can be no obstructions or jamming up. But this ideogram *du* must not be taken too literally because the *si du* (四 瀆), the four *du,* are actually the four great rivers of China. Thus on the massive scale of China these four rivers represent the great movement of irrigation, which is at the same time the movement of free drainage towards the sea. Perhaps in the triple heater we will find this power to ensure that everything communicates well with the sea within the being, and especially with what we call the four seas.

We find this ideogram *du* used again to characterize more particularly the specialized action of the lower heater.

We will see in the Ling shu that the triple heater is connected to the kidneys. As you know, the kidneys are also the power of the origin and contain the origin of the life of a being. They have this double presence of water and fire which are called the authentic water and fire. But this original unity of water and fire within the kidneys renders them imperceptible, and the triple heater is also imperceptible. Fire and water, at the level of the kidneys, are like the primitive and fundamental unity of the living being. It is quite impossible and intangible - without form, but through the triple heater fire and water can produce effects. They do not have a form but there is the possibility of transformation and diffusion which will make all manifestation possible, and possibly the evolution of all the organs, if you are looking at it from a genetic point of view. But that is speculation.

Claude Larre: I think that it is much clearer if we take this not for the human being but for the universe itself. If you take heaven as one part, with earth facing heaven, you find fire and the sun in heaven and water on earth. Therefore there is nothing higher between heaven and earth than fire and water. Then if the human being is just combining heaven's power with earth's ability to receive, it is the fire of heaven and the water of earth which make the human. The triple heater affects this mixing of water and fire in the kidneys. It is easier to understand if you put that which pertains to the triple heater in a broader frame.

Elisabeth Rochat: When Su wen chapter 8 insists on the pathway of liquids and the regulation of fluids it is just to make this action of the triple heater more tangible by means of this image of the movement of liquids inside the body. It makes the links with the kidneys and the water of the kidneys closer. But in order for the liquids to use the pathways there first has to be a strength which is capable of opening these passages and going through them, and afterwards of ensuring that the liquids are in their proper place in each part of the trunk. At each level there are specific organs that are responsible for the regulation of liquids. The role of the triple heater is to ensure that everything circulates harmoniously throughout these levels. It is a kind of regulator which relies on each of the individual functions at the various different levels, but which goes beyond them because it takes account of the whole of the body and being.

Question: Is it concerned with blood?

Elisabeth Rochat: The triple heater is essentially active on the *qi*. The middle heater is the place where the basis for the blood is made, and *qi* is necessary for the circulation of blood. The triple heater is not primarily concerned with blood, but there is never a function which is completely independent of any other, and if the triple heater is really a very primitive intermediary between this being that does not yet have a form and the being which comes about and develops little by little, then it must have a certain influence on the quantity and quality of the blood. But in treatment you would look for the organs that are more immediately responsible, for example the spleen or the liver. You would treat the triple heater much more for the general animation, and for a reestablishment of the unity of communication, circulation and harmonization.

Question: In the embryo which comes first, the organs or the heater?

Elisabeth Rochat: It is really quite impossible to say, but we can speculate on what is one and two and three and four and five! One may be *ming men* (命 門), the representation of the fundamental unity of a new living being. Two could be two kidneys, *yin yang* (陰 陽), fire and water, heaven and earth. We know that *ming men* is between the two kidneys, between the power of the fire and the water and between *yin* and *yang*, two could be the primitive expression in an human being of this duality. Three could be the triple heater, this exchange between the two poles, between *yin* and *yang*, fire and water and so on, this exchange for communication and transformation.

And what of four? We can continue like this, four limbs which are the extension of the form of the body, but there are also the four seas inside the body, or the first of the extraordinary meridians, *du mai, ren mai, chong mai* and *dai mai.* There are five *zang* and six *fu*, and six extraordinary *fu*, and seven orifices. But all this is just speculation through numerology. The problem is that we have no Chinese texts which can answer occidental questions on embryology.

Claude Larre: It is an answer without a question because you must understand that in the Chinese view it is enough to present life as they observe it. The continuity between the universal organization of being and the ability of our mind to understand that only goes to prove that it is the same organization in your mind as in the phenomenon you observe. The only way to understand life is to be conscious of your own life. And when you make an analysis using numbers be aware that numbers are just the reflection of the movement in your own mind. You understand what heaven is doing, but you have to be content with your own knowledge and your knowledge applies only to facts where seen.

I mean that *tian di* (天 地), heaven earth, the universe and your own reflection or action, are not a problem if you observe things as they are. There is no difference between the organization of the universe and the reflection in your mind if your mind is correct, and that is reflected in the Chinese classical language. The mind is just a mirror, so if you see a lot of intricacies here it is because your mind is not able to see in a very simple way how heaven and earth are working. Lao zi chapter 42 talks about all this. So the play of numbers is up to you, but the fact that you understand or do not understand is not due to the numbers but to the selection of numbers that you make.

LING SHU CHAPTER 2

Elisabeth Rochat: It is in the Ling shu that we find most of the information on the triple heater. In Ling shu chapter 2 the different couples of the *zang* with their respective *fu* are presented, for example the lung and the large intestine. When you reach the fifth pair, the kidneys, it says:

> *The kidneys are connected to the bladder, and the bladder is the fu of the liquids, jin ye (津 液), of the body... Shao yang is dependent on the kidneys, the kidneys above are connected to the lungs, and this is why they have a double storage.*

The ideogram for thesaurization or storage is the same ideogram as for organ. It has the idea of actively keeping something very precious, and in this context the something very precious is the essences. So the kidneys have a double storage. The text continues:

> The triple heater is the fu for the irrigation that is in the middle.

The expression is *zhong du* (中 瀆), and *du* is the character that we saw earlier, the canal which represents every kind of current, circulation or communication. When we add this notion of central or median, then this designates the triple heater. The Ling shu continues by saying that the regulation of fluids stems from it which is reminiscent of Su wen chapter 8. The text finishes:

> The triple heater is dependent on the bladder, it is a solitary fu.

So the triple heater as a *fu* is connected to the kidneys because they have a double storage, a double power which is like a couple. Commentators are sometimes more precise about this. They say that the left kidney is joined to the function of the bladder and the right kidney is linked to the triple heater. We know from Nan jing 36 that the left kidney represents the kidneys as the power of water and the function of the bladder, which is in charge of all the liquids in the body, and the right kidney is *ming men,* which is the power of fire at the level of the kidneys. And the link between the triple heater and the fire of *ming men* is repeated in many texts.

Here we find the idea of communication which irrigates and pervades everywhere: it depends on a power which is central and median. It is a mediating power, an intermediary power, an exchanging power, like a go-between. But go-between is not exactly the meaning of *zhong* (中). *Zhong* is central, and central can be median, or in the middle, but it is not exactly a go-between. That would be another ideogram *shi* (使), the ambassador or messenger.

COMMENTARY BY ZHANG JIEBIN

Elisabeth Rochat: Now we will look at the commentary of a great doctor from the beginning of the 17th century, Zhang Jiebin. He says:

> *The triple heater, although it is the fu of all the drainage and irrigation of the middle, is also that which gathers together and protects all the yang.*

That is to say, it does not only have the regulation of fluids under its command, but also the regulation of the *yang,* and it has as its title the fire minister. It is also the *fu* of the fire in the middle of the water, which is a way of indicating that the fire is within the kidneys, the fire of *ming men* between the two kidneys. It is the *yin* power, dependent on the bladder and it connects with the water of the kidneys. Because of this we say the lower heater is like an irrigation canal. So the interpretation of Zhang Jiebin is that it is a *yin* power when it is in a descending movement, and this connects it with the water of the kidneys. Higher up it is *yang* and it connects with *bao luo*, the enveloping network of the heart, and it ensures free communication with the fire of the heart. The text concludes like this:

> *The triple heater, its upper limit and its extreme point below, make it similar to the six reunions or junctions, liu he* (六 合), *of the universe, and there is nothing that it does not envelop or surround.*

The character for reunion, *he* (合), has the mouth radical below to suggest the blowing of breath. The six junctions are above and below the four directions. They are the manner in which the influences of heaven and earth intermingle their qualities and join their *qi* together to form the space in which life can develop.

Claude Larre: Heaven penetrates earth, it has to be outside but inside too. When something is a living being then there is breath, and the *qi* of earth is caused by the pressure of heaven upon earth. When the *qi* of earth manifests we call that the essences. It is important to fix in our minds that *qi* is not the first thing to appear. The first thing to appear is the division inside the unity of heaven and earth, because a combination of heaven and earth is able to produce *qi* for a living being.

Elisabeth Rochat: The six junctions in the human body are formed by the way in which the *jing bie* (經 別), the meridian divergences, join in couples, for example the large intestine with the lungs. The way in which the *qi* of these meridians join together is a way of forming the vital space within the human body, and is related to all the functions of these special pathways detached from the meridians. But this is just an aside!

When we say that the triple heater resembles the six junctions it means that the triple heater is a function which encircles all the living space within a being. This is the interpretation of Ling shu chapter 2 by Zhang Jiebin. What is certain here is that the kidneys have a double storing and are connected on the one hand with the bladder and on the other hand with the *shao yang,* the triple heater.

Why would the text remind us of *shao yang* if not because this young *yang* is the *yang* that is born from the middle of water and can transport the power of the primitive fire. Here we find again that minister fire is linked with *ming men* and with the triple heater, and with all the network of communication around the heart. It is the way in which fire appears and circulates everywhere in the being. This fire is necessary for the proper functioning of each organ. It is said that without the fire of *ming men* no organ could function, or even exist.

This fire minister travels and circulates, rises and falls, ensures all free communication and all the connections and concentrations which can then give the form of life. It is the same as the fire that circulates between heaven and earth and which makes life appear and germinate. So we can understand the deep relationship between the fire of *ming men* (命 門) and the triple heater as this diffusion and blossoming of an efficient and active fire throughout all parts of the individual. We can also understand how *xin zhu* (心 主) and the network of communication of the heart use the same fire minister in order to ensure their function. Here we also have a communication between anterior and posterior heaven, that is between everything that is at the origin of the being and everything that is for the reconstitution of the being in line with these original models.

Therefore in this passage of the Ling shu we have the connection of the triple heater with the kidneys and the bladder, the affirmation that the triple heater ensures the circulation and irrigation of the liquids and *qi* in the body. It is capable of doing this because it takes its strength from the fire of the kidneys, and because it plays the role of an intermediary at every level of life. Fire and water, in a human body as well as in the universe between heaven and earth, freely exchange their full usefulness and efficiency. There is no vital water without fire to transform it and no fire of life without water to fix and express it.

THE TRIPLE HEATER MERIDIAN IN LING SHU CHAPTER 2

Elisabeth Rochat: In this same chapter there is another particular presentation of the triple heater. When the so-called five element points are given for each meridian, the triple heater is treated specially, and in fact is mentioned three times. Here is the text:

> *The triple heater above joins with the shao yang of the hand and comes out at guan chong (關 衝 TH 1), at the extremity of the ring finger. It is the well point and the metal point. It flows down and is the fu of the liquid at ye men (液 門 TH 2), which is the rong (榮) point. It spreads with power to zhong zhu (中 渚 TH 3), in the middle of a hollow, at the rear of the metacarpo-phalangeal joint, the yu (俞) point. It passes to yang chi (陽 池 TH 4), which is in a hollow below the wrist and is the source point. It circulates to zhi gou (支 溝) which is in the hollow between the two bones above the wrist in the*

centre, and is the jing (經) point. It penetrates the depths at tian jing (天 井 TH 10), which is in the hollow above the large bone on the outside of the elbow in the centre. It is the reunion, he (合) point, and you bend the elbow to find it.

The same kind of presentation is made for all the other meridians, but the text for the triple heater continues by saying:

Its yu (俞) point below is at the anterior surface of the big toe, behind the shao yang (少 陽). It comes out on the external surface in the middle of the calf and its name is wei yang (委 陽).

This is Bl 39 in the new numbering system, Bl 53 in the old. It is a network of connection, a *luo* (絡), of the *tai yang* (大 陽). The text continues:

The triple heater is what accompanies shao yang (少 陽) and tai yin (大 陰).

The text here is certainly corrupted, and the majority of commentators correct it. The problem is that they are not in agreement about the correction! Some say the triple heater is what accompanies the *shao yang* (少 陽) and the *tai yang* (大 陽), and others say the triple heater is what accompanies the *shao yin* (少 陰) and the *tai yin* (大 陰). We will look later on at the different possible explanations.

> *It is a detachment, bie* (別)*, of tai yang. At five cun above the malleolus it separates and enters deeply, passing the upper part of the calf. It comes out at wei yang* (委 陽 *Bl 39), (the departure point of the jing bie* (經 別) *of tai yang).*

So the triple heater enters into the depths of the body to take a *luo* (絡) relationship, to connect up, with the bladder. Then there are some clinical symptoms:

> *In case of fullness there is anuria or dysuria. When there is emptiness there is urinary incontinence. In the case of urinary incontinence you tonify and in case of anuria or disuria you sedate (or disperse).*

In this chapter we can see how the triple heater is presented as omnipresent in the body, and not simply reduced to its expression as the *shao yang* of the hand, all of which is exceptional in the framework of these presentations in Ling shu chapter 2.

First there is the presentation of the meridian, then of its junction above, and then below, where the power of the triple heater is rooted right down in the big toe, the big toe serving as a support for the *yin* meridians. Sometimes the text is corrected to the little toe, and in those instances it is the *tai yang* which is more present. Either you see it as drawn from below, rooted downwards into the *yin,* given a great *yin* resonance if it is put with the big toe. Or on the other hand it can be linked to the power of *tai yang* which spreads in the little toe. In any case it is with the *tai yang* that it has a certain communion of *qi* since it is a point on the bladder, *wei yang* (委 陽), which has a special action on the triple heater and is given as its *yu* point below.

The triple heater is linked to *tai yang* in the same way as if it were a *luo* connection in this region of the popliteal crease. At the point *wei yang* it is possible to regulate the triple heater and influence its rooting towards the bottom. It is always said to be the lower *he* point of the triple heater, as if it were a point where you could grasp the power of the triple heater through the *tai yang* and the bladder. This comes back to what we were saying earlier, that the triple heater is dependent on the bladder, particularly for everything that is for drainage below.

Thirdly and finally there is a presentation in the text which concerns the central region of the body. Here the triple heater is seen as the intermediary between the *tai yang* and *shao yang* of the leg. This is understandable because being the *shao yang* of the hand it shares the same quality of *qi* as the *shao yang* of the foot, the gallbladder, and it has a privileged connection with *tai yang* because of its special relationship with the bladder, and with the kidneys because the bladder and triple heater are both special *fu* of the kidneys. In this third presentation the triple heater either accompanies the *shao yin* or the *tai yang* in which case it is found between the bladder and the kidneys. But it particularly follows the pathway of the *jing bie* of *tai yang* that penetrates the lower abdomen. This very close connection of the bladder and the lower heater regulates the elimination of liquids: this is seen pathologically as either anuria or dysuria if there is too great a pressure forcing the liquids out in too great a quantity, or incontinence which is a loosening preventing tension and retention. The symptoms, in this latter case, follow the model of the pathology of the great *luo, da luo* (大 絡), in Ling shu chapter 10.

We have here, therefore, a triple presentation of the triple heater which is anchored above at the extremity of the ring finger, and which is rooted below in the big toe, or just in the toes in general, the text is not clear on this. But what is clear is that it is rooted in the toes which are the lower extremity of the body, and this gives a particular connection between the *qi* of leg *tai yang* and the *qi* of *shao yang*, a connection which can be particularly grasped at the point *wei yang*, Bl 53, and finally which manifests inside the body in the proper regulation of the outflow of liquids.

The kidneys are well served by this union of bladder and triple heater, and in particular the lower heater. We have to remember the two sides of the two aspects of the lower heater: all the direction and drainage of liquids on one hand, and the fire of *ming men* (命 門) and the lower cinnabar field (*dan tian* 丹 田) on the other. The fire and cinnabar field permit all the transformations of *qi*. This is mentioned in Su wen chapter 8 where the bladder is said to control and store all the liquids in the body and then, through the transformations of *qi*, enable all the manifestations of power. It is by means of this alliance, this close connection, that the relationship of the bladder and triple heater is maintained. And what is interesting is that the pathology of the triple heater is clearly linked to the lower part of the body.

LING SHU CHAPTER 18

Huang di asked Qi Bo: How does man receive qi?
How do yin and yang join together (hui 會)?
What qi forms the basis of vital nutrition (ying 營)?
What qi forms the defence (wei 衛)?
From where is the nutritive produced and how?
Where and how do the joining together (hui) for defence take place?

The old and the strong (those in the prime of life) do not have the same qi, yin and yang do not have the same positions. I would like to be instructed on all that!

Qi Bo replied: Man receives qi from the cereals. The cereals enter the stomach to be transmitted to the lung. The five zang and six fu will all receive this qi. Those that are clear produce the ying. Those that are unclear produce the wei. The nutritive qi circulates within the mai (脈). The defensive qi circulates outside the mai. The nutritive qi runs its circuit without stopping; 50 times and there is once again a great reunion. Yin and yang interlink and interconnect like a circle without end.

The defensive qi circulates 25 times in the yin and 25 times in the yang; they are divided according to the day and night. So it is that when the qi reaches the yang there is activity and when the qi reaches the yin there is rest.

This is why it is said: in the middle of the day the yang is in the position of the eminent dragon (long 龍), and that makes the redoubled yang (zhong yang 重陽). In the middle of the night the yin is in the position of the eminent dragon and that makes the redoubled yin (zhong yin 重陰).

So it is that tai yin governs the interior and tai yang governs the exterior. Each circulates 25 times, the division being made according to day and night. In the middle of the night it is the redoubled yin; after the middle of the night it is the declining yin (yin shuai 陰衰); at dawn the yin reaches its end and the yang receives the qi. In the middle of the day it is the redoubled yang; at the end of the afternoon it is the declining yang (yang shuai 陽 衰); at sunset the yang reaches its end and the yin receives the qi.

In the middle of the night is a great reunion, everyone is asleep. The usual expression is reunion in the yin (he yin 合 陰). At dawn when the yin draws to its end and the yang receives qi without interruption, this is done in the image of the ordered unfolding of heaven and earth.

Huang di: When old men do not sleep at night, which qi is responsible? When strong men do not sleep in the day, which qi is responsible?

Qi Bo: As for strong men, their qi and blood are in full power (sheng 盛), their flesh is oily, their qi flows freely (qi dao tong 氣 道 通), the circulations of nutrition and defence occur normally; this is why they are full of life (jing 精) in the day and they sleep well at night.

As for old men, their qi and blood are in decline (shuai 衰) their flesh dries out, their qi flows with difficulty, the qi of the five zang fight with each other, their nutritive qi declines and becomes scarce while their defensive qi is drained on the inside. This is why they are lifeless (bu jing 不 精), in the day and they do not sleep at night.

Huang di: I would like to know about the circulations of nutrition and defence; through what pathways do they arrive?

Qi Bo replied: That which nourishes (ying 營) comes out of the middle heater. That which defends (wei 衛) comes out of the lower heater.

Huang di: I would like to know where the three heaters (san jiao 三 焦) come out (chu 出).

Qi Bo replied: The upper heater (shang jiao 上 焦) comes out at the upper mouth of the stomach; it joins with the pharynx rising and entering the diaphragm and diffusing in the middle of the thorax (xiong zhong 胸 中). It reaches the axilla and proceeds following the division of the area of tai yin; returning, it reaches the yang ming, rises to attain the tongue and descends to the yang ming of the foot.

Its normal circulation is with the nutritive (ying 營); 25 times in the yang, 25 times in the yin, which makes one circuit. So every 50 times, there is a return to the great reunion (da hui 大 會) in the tai yin of the hand.

Huang di: When man is overheated and the liquid and solid food descend to the stomach, the qi is unstable and sweat comes out; it comes out either on the face or on the back or on one side of the body; it does not come out following the pathways of the defensive qi. Why?

Qi Bo: In this case there is an external injury by wind; from the interior there is an opening of the cou li (腠 理) the body hairs being impregnated with vapour, there is a flowing out from the lineaments (cou li 腠 理). The defensive qi runs there. Because of this, of course it cannot follow its pathways. This qi is alive and fiery, slippery and quick, meeting with an opening, it comes out. It is for this reason that it cannot follow its pathways; and this is why the usual name given is loss by flowing out (lou xie 漏 泄).

Huang di: I would like to know where the middle heater comes out.

Qi Bo replied: The middle heater (zhong jiao 中 焦) is also associated with the middle of the stomach (in another version: the mouth of the stomach). It comes after the upper heater. It receives qi, filters (mi 泌) the residues and waste (zao po 糟 粕) vapourizes (zheng 蒸) the interstitial fluids (jin ye (津 液) transforms (hua 化) the jing wei (精 微) rises and spreads out in the mai (脈) of the lungs; and there is transformation into blood, bringing life to the body. Nothing is more precious. It is because of this that it alone can circulate in the channels of the

meridians (jing sui 經 隧)the usual term is nutritive qi
(ying qi 營 氣)...

Huang di: Blood (xue 血)and qi, under different names
(ming 名)are of the same type (lei 類). How is this?

Qi Bo replied: Nutrition and defence (ying wei 營 衛) are
essences and qi (jing qi 精 氣). Blood is spirits and qi
(shen qi 神 氣). It is for this reason that blood and qi
have different names while being of the same type. When
one loses blood, there is no sweat and when one loses
sweat, there is no blood. So it is that human life, which
has two deaths, does not have two lives.

Huang di: I would like to know where the lower heater
comes out.

Qi Bo replied: The lower heater (xia jiao 下 焦) separates
(bie 別) at the turning intestine, spreads to the bladder
where it enters through infiltration (shen 滲). It belongs
to the liquids and cereals associated with the stomach
which they occupy to constitute the residues and dregs
which descend to the large intestine; and that makes up
the lower heater. By infiltration everything descends; it
favours the passage which, through filtering, separates
the juices which follow the lower heater to enter the
bladder by infiltration.

Huang di: When one drinks alcohol, alcohol enters the stomach. Why then, before the cereals have been cooked by digestion (shu 熟) is there a descent of urine?

Qi Bo replied: Alcohol is liquid (ye 液) from cooked cereals (shu gu 熟 穀). Its qi is bold and clear (qing 清). This is why, even though it entered after the cereals, this liquid comes out before them.

Huang di: Very good. I now know that the upper heater is like a mist (wu 霧) that the middle heater is like a maceration (ou 漚) and that the lower heater is like a canal (du 瀆).

Elisabeth Rochat: The title of Ling shu chapter 18 is Ying wei sheng hui (營 衛 生 會). That is to say, how that which nourishes and deeply organizes the being which we call the nutritive energy, the *ying* (營), and that which animates and defends this organized life, the wei (衛), come together, join and meet. And this chapter presents us with some of the most ancient and some of the best definitions of each of the three heaters.

It is interesting that its title is not the definitive description of the three heaters, but simply of the nature of nutritive and defensive *qi*. When we consider the way they are produced and the way they can circulate harmoniously (that is the way they come together and function in the same living being) then we see that in fact the three heaters are all that allows transformation and circulation, and gathers together the particular work of each organ. It is from this gathering together that the *ying* and the *wei* are produced. It is also traditionally said that nutrition comes from the middle heater, and that defensive energy comes from the upper or lower heater, depending on the context.

Question: Is there any relevance in practice to the fact that it circulates 25 times in the day and 25 times at night?

Elisabeth Rochat: It is difficult to say. You can try to make pictures or tables but I am not sure if that actually leads to anything. It is above all the idea of an equilibrium which is extraordinarily well balanced and which is not just an internal equilibrium but which is balanced with all the cycles which make the universe. But whether the fact that it is 25 and 25 is relevant to practice, I am not sure.

Claude Larre: Perhaps what is more relevant is the balance between the nutritive and defensive within the day. When we feel in very good condition, we feel at the same time that we are able to counter attack of any sort, and that if an effort is needed then we are able to make it because the nourishment has been good enough. Perhaps the feeling of quietness and strength is given by the *sheng hui* (生 會), the meeting of the forces of life which determine that we have enough reserves to nourish ourselves, and enough power to counter attack. This could be further realised in the balance between the *ying* and the *wei.*

Elisabeth Rochat: There are commentaries on these questions of the circulation of nutritive and defensive *qi* in the body, and there are other chapters in the Ling shu that take up the problem of the circulation of the different energies again, and they link them with the rhythm of respiration. In respiration there is usually a kind of regular progression, and this is linked to the general circulation of the meridians. This falls back on the circulation of the nutrition in the meridians, 25 times in the day and 25 times at night. So it is a circulation which is just as regular as breathing itself, and which is carried on very regularly.

The defensive *qi* is not the same since its circulation is much freer and it goes everywhere. Regarding the practical application of this we will come back to the symptoms later.

THE UPPER HEATER
SHANG JIAO

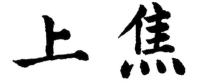

Elisabeth Rochat: One of the great functions of the upper heater is to gather together the heart, the lung and the sea of *qi*, to bring together the beating of the heart, the rhythm of respiration and the sea of *qi* out of which everything that circulates in the body can spring. That is the nutritive and the defensive *qi*. This is what the upper heater really is - the synthesis of everything which makes the *qi* circulate and pulsate rhythmically. This is explained in the definition given by Qi Bo when he says it is in the upper part of the trunk at the upper mouth of the stomach. Why should there be mention of this if not to remind us that the upper heater also has this function of introducing something into the organism. It has mastery over the entry ways and over what is introduced, and when Qi Bo mentions the pharynx he is referring to the arrival of all the food that comes into the stomach.

Afterwards he says that it rises and diffuses in the middle of the thorax, and this is in order to pass onto the next stage, because when we speak of the three heaters, when something is introduced it is in order to be transformed. Since we are in the upper heater the final outcome of this transformation is the purified *qi* which rises up above the thorax and forms the sea of *qi* in the chest.

It is at this point that certain commentators say that the upper heater is *tan zhong* (膻 中). We saw previously the close connection between *tan zhong* and *xin bao luo* (心 包 絡). For example, if you look at the pathway of the *shao yang* of the hand, the triple heater meridian, as it is given in Ling shu chapter 10, it begins at the end of the ring finger, goes up the arm and enters the region of Stomach 12 which is a very important crossroads. The *qi* of *shao yang* spreads out at *tan zhong* and then diffuses and takes a connecting (*luo* 絡) relationship with *xin bao* (心 包), the envelopes or membranes around the heart. Then it descends through the diaphragm and takes a relationship of dependence with each of the three heaters. So in this pathway we see that the meridian of the triple heater takes a particular relationship with *tan zhong* on one hand and with *xin bao* on the other. These are all closely linked because *tan zhong* and *xin bao* are both messengers and ministers for the heart, although *tan zhong* relates specifically to the *qi* and the place where the ancestral *qi* is stored. After all, what is the ancestral *qi* (*zong qi* 宗 氣) if not the way to conserve all the *qi* which is produced by the body in a unity, by means of which the body can continue to live.

Claude Larre: If I may say all this in a simpler manner, everything that makes up the unity of life reminds us of our ancestors. I have no power in myself to be a particular being if that is not related to the fact that I am the descendent of an ancestor. This collective power to make the togetherness of self is something which comes from the fact that I am the son of somebody. And the image for that old, old *qi* is the sea, the sea of *qi*. But when we see this same *qi* actively distributed throughout all the different processes that are required for making life, then we no longer think of it as the sea of *qi*, but as distinct streams of *qi* moving here and there and doing what they have to do.

So the definition of *tan zhong* (膻 中) is really very close to the sea of *qi*, and I would prefer to make *tan zhong*, the sea of *qi* and the ancestors into one unit related to life before me and in me, and as a guiding line for the organization of my own personality.

Elisabeth Rochat: I would remind you that it is the *zong qi* (宗 氣) that makes the heart beat, and it is the *zong qi* that makes the breathing work. So *zong qi* is a power that enables things to move and at the same time remain in a family-like relationship.

Claude Larre: The clanship of the Chinese is surely reflected in this concept of life, where there is a congregation of many people under the protection of a single house and all under the protective influence of the ancestor.

Elisabeth Rochat: In the texts of the Ling shu there is usually no talk of circulation of *zong qi* but rather of accumulation, and even this accumulation is not in the sense of something piling up.

Question: Tan zhong, the point in the centre of the chest, (Ren 17) is forbidden to needle in some schools. Is that because of the risk of dissipating that accumulation?

Claude Larre: In going to the origin, if it is not done correctly, one might lose the origin, and what happens to life then? The more useful things are, the less we can use them because they are so dangerous!

Question: Is there a particular significance in the fact that it says the *tai yin* cannot really be diminished?

Elisabeth Rochat: Yes, of course. I think the explanation is quite easy because the circulation of the nutritive *ying qi* is more internal. Animation begins with the lung meridian, *tai yin* of the hand, and the circulation of the more external, defensive *wei qi* is connected with *tai yang* of the foot, the bladder meridian. Another explanation is that *tai yin* is the maximum *yin* and is the element of the humus, the soil, the earth. *Tai yang* is the more external circulation of the *qi.*

Once you have defined the upper heater as the starting place for the diffusion of all *qi*, then you have a model for this nutritive circulation. Obviously the defensive *qi* will also have its own particular circulation, and we have defined its pathway as starting from the eye with the bladder meridian. But it is not exactly a pathway. When we talk about the circuits of the *ying* and *wei* it is better to see them as moments of intensity rather than like a train leaving a station at a particular time, and arriving at another station at another time.

Of course at every place and at every moment there is nutrition and there is defence. But the *ying* and the *wei* emanate from the upper heater because it is there that they converge before following their own particular destinies. Also there are defensive energies that circulate everywhere around the meridians and in the *luo* (絡). They are pulsated by the same movement that pulsates the nutritive energy, but there is also a circuit of defensive energy which maintains the equilibrium of the person between day and night.

THE MIDDLE HEATER
ZHONG JIAO

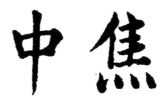

Elisabeth Rochat: The middle heater is associated with the middle of the stomach. Here you will notice that we are at the second of the four seas, since we had the sea of *qi* in the middle of the chest, and we have here the heart of the stomach which is the sea of liquids and cereals. The stomach has one of the most important functions in the body, being the ability to extract from food that which will constitute the body. This explains why the middle heater is associated with the middle of the stomach. It receives the *qi,* it filters the residues and wastes, vapourizes the *jin ye* (津 液), and transforms the *jing wei (*精 微), and this is a whole group of functions which go beyond the stomach and which constitute this process of extraction from food. There is a filtration of all that will continue to descend, and the end of this process in the intestines will give the excrement.

It also vapourizes the *jin ye* (津 液). That is to say there is something like an emission of vapour or steam, a very humid vapour, which rises and forms very pure liquids which are full of life, and capable of passing throughout the whole organism to irrigate it, and also to rinse it out. So the *jin ye* have to be charged with all that is essential for life, and they must be very light and airy. Then it says it transforms the *jing wei* (精 液). We have seen this expression several times before. The *jing* are the essences, and the *wei* are something very subtle and almost imperceptible. So what is the transformation related to the *jing wei*? It is to take the food which arrives in the stomach with its own essences and flavour and vital elements which do not belong to you, and to make them into your life. To do this you have to atomize them in some way, reduce them to a state which is so broken up, so decomposed and so fine that they can penetrate your structure. That is what this ideogram *wei* signifies in this context. It is the transformation of those essences that do not belong to you being turned into essences which can be yours. And what are your own essences if not the vital elements from the exterior, recomposed in the fundamental model of composition, the first compenetration which brought you into life, and which later on are called the essences of anterior heaven.

The essences in oneself are the model of composition and recomposition of what makes your life, and in this lies the importance of the middle heater which perpetually recomposes your own vitality from exterior elements. This vitality will appear again under the aspect of blood which is formed thanks to the work of the middle heater from the essences, the juices and the liquids which become your own and which are charged with the vitality that you assimilate and what passes from the middle heater to the upper heater. It is here that the *mai* (脈) of the lungs is connected. You already know that the lung meridian begins in the middle heater, that it descends and then rises up again, and when it reaches the upper heater there is a transformation which creates blood.

There are very rich liquids which come from the middle heater pure enough to pass through the barrier of the diaphragm, which are presented to the field of oxygenation in the lungs, and then - and we know this from different texts - to the heart. And it is the heart that makes the final transformation and gives the inspiration of the spirits to this liquid, the mark and seal of which is the red colour. The specificity of blood in relation to other liquids is that it is the only one which, coming from the middle heater, needs the action of the upper heater in order to be what it is. It is for this reason that the blood is a liquid quite different from the others in Chinese medicine. The nutrition that it brings the body is more than just a simple maintenance. It is that which makes life itself, that which gives the inspiration of the spirits. It is because of this that it says in the text that the blood brings life to the body, and in this text each word is weighted.

So we have the presence of the essences coming from the middle heater, and the presence of the spirits which are in the heart. That is to say that in the blood we have the action of the essences and the spirits. There is the pulsing of the blood by the *qi,* but what this *qi* pulsates or moves is not just the simple nutrition of the body, it is the circulation of the spirits themselves. It is the influence of the spirits which gives us both the similarity and the difference between the construction or nutrition of the being and the blood.

This is what is explained in the sentence:

> *Nutrition and defence are essences and qi, blood is spirits and qi.*

Obviously the connections are very close since there is a nutrition and a building of the being which is also made by the blood. The blood is totally interlinked with the proper functioning of the middle heater because if there is not enough basis to present to the heart for transformation, then the spirits will never have a place through which to transmit their influence, and the blood will be poor and deficient. The root and foundation of the blood are in the middle heater.

THE LOWER HEATER
XIA JIAO

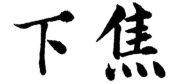

Elisabeth Rochat: So we reach the lower heater which is seen in Ling shu chapter 18 in its role as a canal for drainage, for separating and descending the residue and waste. It directs liquids towards the bladder where the penetration is made through some kind of osmosis or filtration, because the Chinese knew very well that there was no strict anatomical orifice connecting the bladder with the small intestine. All the liquids are led to the field of action of the bladder, and here there is purification and recovery of that which can still be useful. When you purify these unclear liquids they regain their original form and their ability to ascend in the form of mists and vapours. All the liquids from the drainage and rinsing will make up the urine, and all the substances that continue to dry out and will finally end up as excrement are directed towards the large intestine.

Here we have all that constitutes the lower heater, the good regulation of everything which must be eliminated, and that which must be recuperated. But of course there is also the presence of fire in the lower heater, which allows everything that may still be useful to rise up in the form of a mist. In order for there to be circulation in the trunk there has to be a fire below to stimulate this upward movement, just as there has to be a fire in the centre of the chest to govern the movement of diffusion. This is all part of the lower heater. And when it is said that the defensive *qi* comes from the lower heater, it is because it is enriched in some way and marked by this lower fire. It is this that gives the defensive *qi* its very lively aspect and which allows it to fulfil its function of defence.

Question: I do not understand why the defensive *qi* comes from the lower heater?

Elisabeth Rochat: It is because there is a continuation of descent from the middle heater. All the usefulness has not been taken out of the food by the middle heater so there is a further extraction and refining, and above all a transformation at the level of the lower heater. This is why it is said that the clear is linked with the nutritive *qi* and the unclear is linked with the defensive. At first this seems bizarre because that which is clear is that which is animated with movement and with the *yang* and which rises the most, and what is called unclear is that which is most dense and most stable and interior. So there is a contradiction here. What is indicated is that the defensive *qi* comes from the lower heater from that which has continued to descend and which is more dense and which cannot take this aspect of defence and *yang* energy except through the action of *ming men* and the fire in the lower heater. It is a bit like coal. Coal is unclear, it is black and it is dense, but if you set fire to it then you have a completely different effect. This is a parallel image. So in order for there to be defence in the organism there has to be participation from this deepest fire within the being, and the fire of *ming men* (命 門) has to be fully expressed in the defensive *qi.*

From this we can see that the triple heater propagates *qi* everywhere but is in particular the agent for the distribution of original *qi* which comes from *ming men.* It is because of this that it is sometimes said that the defensive *qi* comes from the upper heater and sometimes from the lower heater. You either take the origin as the place in which they are formed or the place where they are distributed. What we have to understand from all this is that both for the nutritive and for the defensive *qi* it is the free circulation and the working together, the collaboration of all the organs which is in fact called the triple heater. We will also see later on that the triple heater is a continual intermediary between the organs, the origin and what is reconstituted on this model.

Question: If you need the essences from food for the *qi* of life how do people fast? If you have to have *qi* for life, fasting is not actually having any essences coming through the stomach for a long time.

Elisabeth Rochat: If one lacks food and cannot sustain one's vitality because there is not enough basis from which the *qi* can emerge, then this is a pathological state of weakness which can continue until death. But we can also see there are spiritual people who just eat three grains of rice a day. So what does that mean? In my opinion it means that they know how not to waste. They can draw their life from very little because they really know how to extract all the life that this small quantity contains, and they know how to regulate their *qi* and how to conduct and direct the *qi* within themselves. Perhaps they know a lot of Daoist exercises, meditations and visualizations for example, so they know how to breathe and think and act without being too disturbed.

Claude Larre: They can effect all the necessary transformations without any loss of their energy, like a well-oiled machine. So if we are able to impose conditions of minimum expenditure on the way we are using up the resources in the natural world there is no reason why we should not apply the same doctrine to our own consumption of what is necessary for individual life.

Elisabeth Rochat: What is necessary, in fact, is to make no effort. If we look at the term *yi* (易) mutation or change, as in the Yi jing, the Book of Changes, it also has the meaning of ease, to do something easily, because natural change must be made without effort and without loss. So if someone goes on a fast but does not at the same time have a well-regulated physical, spiritual and mental life, they will probably become ill. But it is possible that through the extraordinary action of the spirits your needs diminish so you do not waste your *qi* and you can make less effort.

Question: Can the ill be similarly helped to recovery by the utilization of spiritual energies?

Elisabeth Rochat: You cannot recover unless you have a good frame of mind and a good mental and spiritual condition. Either you put yourself in a certain axis or current of life, or you completely refuse to be placed in it. And if the patient refuses, you can stick needles in him for ten years and it will not do any good. This is the inner condition of being. But you cannot say you just take a little bit of spiritual energy in order to replace something here. It does not happen like that.

Claude Larre: It might be true sometimes that if a man has enough reserves, going to a musical performance or a good movie, he would have no need of supper, just because being in a very high mental condition he could draw from his own reserves what was necessary to replace the small amount dissipated at the time when he was not eating.

Elisabeth Rochat: But if you have dissipated your reserves it is because you had the wrong frame of mind to start with. It can happen that a saint dies of hunger, but it is not the same thing. He will not have dissipated anything, it is just the circumstances of life. I remember one time there was a friend who came to me with toothache and she wanted me to needle her to relieve the pain. So I did an experiment. This was someone who was in a good state of mind, and I gave her two or three chapters of Lao zi to read and she was very enthusiastic. After a while I asked about her teeth. She had completely forgotten about them and did not have any pain! You can do that with friends, but it is difficult to ask for money for it! And, of course, in the case of an abscess the pain will start again soon.

Question: On this same idea of fasting, would you say that somewhere there is the idea that in fasting you are using up waste that has not been correctly eliminated, even if you are not in a particularly spiritual frame of mind. Is there a possibility that you are still producing a kind of cleansing process?

Elisabeth Rochat: Fasts can have this effect, but if someone just stops eating for a certain time and then goes back into a kind of regular life I wonder if it actually has much effect.

Claude Larre: It might be that during the time of fasting the *po* (魄) are free to work with the waste. If you are eating and drinking too much and are overdoing it, then the *po* do not have enough time to dispose of the waste. But if you fast then they have more time to get rid of the excess. Then I am quite sure your assumption has some basis.

Elisabeth Rochat: If you just stop eating because of an idea or a fashion it will not last as an effect. But if you go on a fast in order to try and transform, then it will have a much more long-lasting effect, and through this rest you can unblock something.

THE TRIPLE HEATER AS A MIST, A MACERATION AND A DRAINAGE CANAL

Elisabeth Rochat: We will continue with the three descriptions of the three heaters as a mist, a maceration and a canal for drainage, *wu* (霧), *ou* (漚) and *du* (瀆). As we saw before there is the idea of water and of humidity and dampness in each of these three ideograms. In the last two, *ou* and *du*, we see the three drops of water on the left of the ideograms, and in the first, *wu*, water is present in the form of small drops of rain under the heavenly vault (*yu* 雨). So these three names are very clear in relation to the definitions we saw earlier.

THE UPPER HEATER AS A MIST

Elisabeth Rochat: What is a mist? It is not the mist or fog that makes you cough or wrap up well. This mist suggests everything that rises up from the earth in the form of vapour or steam which is capable of permeating everywhere. This means that at the level of the upper heater, above the diaphragm which is some kind of filter, there are never water or currents of water, but only that which can rise up as misty vapour. Everything which has managed to cross the filter of the diaphragm from the middle heater is then able to pervade the whole body like some kind of mist. So it is everything we have seen in the circulation of *qi*, the propagation and diffusion from the upper heater reaching the most external parts of the body right up to the skin and body hair, but which also penetrates the bones and flesh just like a vapour.

In this respect the mist exemplifies what we have been saying about the defensive *qi* filling the skin, making the layers of the flesh firm, the structure of the body sound and its functioning smooth. Mist in Chinese thought is that which is subtle and pure enough to rise from the earth and meet the *qi* of heaven, so that in this meeting life can germinate. And the opposite movement of heaven would be the dew which sprinkles the earth.

Mirroring these actions you can see the physiology of the

lung and the relationship between the spleen and the lung through *tai yin* which makes all the subtle *qi* rise from the middle to the upper heater. You can also see how the lung, which is the heaven of the trunk and the five *zang* and six *fu*, makes all the liquids in the body descend throughout the body like some kind of dew. This is just to show that the physiological functions of the human being are exactly the same as the meteorological movements of life in the universe which create clouds and rain and so on, just seen on different levels.

Claude Larre: There is another particular point which is that we can observe that a mist from outside can affect the body with a destructive force, and that hot steam is destructive of the strength of the muscles. We know that in cooking one has to simmer certain sorts of dishes for a long time so that the penetration takes place slowly and perfectly everywhere. Then when we chew what we have prepared it is less tough, and has been well prepared for assimilation.

Elisabeth Rochat: When we were talking about the liquids moving downwards like dew, all of them will finally arrive in the field of action of the bladder in order to be purified or eliminated. Here again we find the ensemble of the three heaters required for the circulation of liquids which takes place in the body. But if we come back to this image of a mist, the upper heater is concerned with the action of diffusion, and that which moves like vapour able to impregnate everything everywhere.

THE MIDDLE HEATER AS A MACERATION

Elisabeth Rochat: This word maceration is not very clear. If you take some kind of receptacle or bowl, and you put food into it, and then add water, if there is ambient heat (because after all this is the middle heater) then it will be soaked and softened and decomposed, and will start to rot a little bit. This is what maceration is. Can anyone think of a better word?

Comment: No. Maceration is a very good word. When you put papaya leaves on steak you are tenderizing it, and that is maceration. If you put any food in wine or vinegar it is also separating fibres. It is any process that breaks down the intactness of the material.

Elisabeth Rochat: In the middle heater the food has already been eaten, so what is necessary is that it has to be assimilated by the stomach and spleen through this kind of humidity or dampness which is full of heat, but which has a fine balance between the dry and the damp, the hot and the cold, so that all these transformations can be made leading to the production of the *jin ye* (津 液).

Claude Larre: I think we are right to come back to this

word maceration since it is a specific Chinese character and not *hua* (化) or *xiao hua* (消 化). *Xiao hua* is digestion, and *hua* is transformation.

Another very important point is that in *wu* (霧), the mist, the water radical is at the top of the character, where the water is part of a working mist to give the power of life in the upper part. In *ou* (漚), maceration, it is on the side, and the disposition of the three squares on the right of the character give the impression of the earth and everything being well disposed in the right place in order to be submitted to the effect of the separation which is made by water, provided some heat is added.

Elisabeth Rochat: All the functions of the stomach and spleen, digestion and assimilation, are seen in this term maceration.

THE LOWER HEATER AS A CANAL

Elisabeth Rochat: Moving on to the lower heater, it is described as a canal, *du* (瀆). We have studied this ideogram already. It is all the flowing and circulation of the liquids with evacuation on one hand and irrigation on the other. It is all the good directing and governing of the liquids in the body, and the separation of the clear and the unclear, and of all that which should be full of humidity and dampness from that which should not. Of course, if you look at the last charges described in Ling shu chapter 18, in particular those of the triple heater, the large intestine and the bladder, you will see that almost all the *zang fu* are involved in this work. So the triple heater is never an isolated function, it is a gathering of all the physiological functions rooted in the original *qi*. We will see this later on in the Nan jing particularly.

The triple heater also relies on the reconstitution of the *qi* and essences in the stomach. It gathers together the original *qi* and the reconstituted *qi*, and makes them work together and circulate everywhere. And it does this in order that all the physiological functions of the *zang fu* function correctly.

LING SHU CHAPTER 30

Elisabeth Rochat: There are many texts which say that the triple heater holds all the *qi* under its authority. And obviously it sees that everything is transformed harmoniously at every moment. But there are other texts in the Ling shu which give us brief descriptions of the heaters, and especially of the upper and middle heaters. For example Ling shu chapter 30. The emperor asks Qi Bo, 'What is qi?' And this is the reply of Qi Bo:

The upper heater makes the opening and outpouring,

disseminates the flavours of the five cereals, diffuses the skin, gives the strength of fullness to the body, keeps the (body) hair oily, irrigates like a mist and a dew. This is called qi (氣). The upper heater makes the opening and outpouring, disseminates the flavours of the five cereals.

Elisabeth Rochat: This means that the essentials which have risen from the middle heater to the upper heater will, in the specific form of the five flavours, be diffused in the five *zang*, and rcvitalized. That is to say the five flavours are a way of seeing the essences which looks at the vital movement that each is most apt to reinforce, for example is it a movement that rises or descends.

'Diffuses the skin' means that it impregnates the layers of the skin as only smoke is capable of doing. It penetrates every space and can go everywhere. If you have a problem with your fireplace then you have smoke everywhere in the house, it is the same idea. You can see the relationship between these two images of mist and smoke, and the idea that they can fill every part of the skin. The word diffuse in English does not give the right feel. In French the word is smoke, but the meaning is lost in my English.

Gives the strength and fullness to the body, keeps the (body) hair oily, irrigates like a mist and a dew, this is called qi.

Here you see all the effects of nutrition and defence through the proper circulation of *qi* as it is defined just by looking at the functions of the upper heater.

A little further on in this same chapter, the Emperor, who is never short of questions, asks, 'What is blood?' And Qi Bo replies:

The middle heater receives qi and grasps the juices...

The ideogram for juices, *zhi* (汁), is made up of water with the number ten, indicating that everything from heaven as well as earth is put together in a perfect unity. So these juices are full of vitality and because of this they can serve as the basis of blood. Therefore when we speak of blood, the middle heater is involved because it is the middle heater that can best extract the vitality which characterizes it.

The upper heater is for the diffusion, the *qi* and the circulation, the middle heater is for the extraction of the essences and the basis for the reconstruction of life, and the lower heater on one hand evacuates the useless, and on the other is the fire which is hidden in the depths and which makes everything simmer and rise up. In this chapter, the upper and middle heaters are used in the definition of *qi* and blood, alluding to the basic couple: blood and *qi.*

LING SHU CHAPTER 81

Elisabeth Rochat: Ling shu chapter 81 says something very similar:

> *The upper heater makes the qi come out in order to warm up the divisions of the flesh.*

Question: What word do they use for the divisions of the flesh?

Elisabeth Rochat: Fen rou (分 肉). It is all the flesh, but considered as muscular masses which are separated or distinguished from one another, and which give the idea of ravines and valleys and the possibility for circulation. The most gross image is that of muscular masses, but within each muscle there is that which allows the possibility of circulation in all the spaces. In each little piece of flesh the *qi* can weave its way through. The flesh is not just a compact mass, but has the capacity to be infiltrated by *qi.* The Chinese always think like this, they are obsessed with the idea of movement.

So the upper heater makes the *qi* circulate in order to warm up these divisions of the skin that we talked about, the *fen rou,* to nourish the bony articulations, and be in free communication with the *cou li* (腠 理).

The middle heater makes the qi come out like a dew.

The dew is already a nutritive liquid which has come from heaven, as opposed to the mist which is a vapour.

They rise to pour out in the large and small valleys, and they infiltrate the most fine and subtle pathways of animation, the mai (脈), right up to the finest pathway.

That is to say everywhere, not just in the meridians, but in every possible place.

The jin ye (津 液), body liquids, are in complete harmony, there are changes and transformations, (bian hua 變化). It is red and that makes the blood.

So there, just in slightly different terms, we have the same ideas.

TRIPLE HEATER AND GALLBLADDER

Elisabeth Rochat: There are a lot of things we can say about this, coming not exactly from the Nei jing or the Nan jing but from later texts.

The *shao yang* is ministerial fire, and *shao yang* is the fire which is rising up from the water, from the depths of life and the kidneys and the origin of life and so on. A later metaphor is of a dragon rising from the water in order to become a dragon flying the skies. So *shao yang* through the gallbladder and the triple heater is the intermediary between these two states of fire and the unfolding of life.

You know that the nature of the *qi* of *shao yang* is to be very great in concentrated strength, but also to be half internal, half external, and to be a mediator, and the gallbladder and triple heater have this common quality of *qi*, each acting in its own way.

Claude Larre: I think there is more to say about the fact that the gallbladder meridian has so many points on it. Is there any truth in the idea that there may be so many points on the gallbladder meridian for the purposes of general distribution, as contrasted with the triple heater which is more for a sort of inspiration?

Elisabeth Rochat: What is certain is that the gallbladder is linked with the essences. Since it is an extraordinary *fu* it stores the essential and pure juices, so it is very much involved in the thesaurization of the essences, while the triple heater is an intermediary or a mediator at every level.

THE TRIPLE HEATER AND THE COU LI

Elisabeth Rochat: Another example is found in Ling shu chapter 47 where we see that the kidneys connect with both the triple heater and the bladder. It is also said here that the triple heater and bladder have their correspondence or their resonance in the *cou li* (腠 理). If we look at the correspondences of all the different *fu* with parts of the body, it says the large intestine corresponds to the skin, the small intestine with the network of animation, the *mai*, the gallbladder with the musculature and the stomach with the flesh. It also notes the correspondences of the *zang* with different parts of the body, for example the kidneys with the bones, the most internal and firm part of the body. And it states that the bladder and the triple heater have their correspondence or resonance in the most external structure of the body, the *cou li.*

The idea of structure is given by this term *li* (理). It is the idea of visible veins in marble, jade or wood. That is to say the very intimate structure of something being manifest in something visible. In other words the very visibility of these veins in wood or stone is just an indication of the real constitution. From this we can see the meaning of this ideogram *li,* the profound, deep structuring, the vital, intimate organization which extends right up to the point of being the natural reason for something. It is like the principle of human intelligence and understanding to have the capacity of perceiving in things and beings their reason for being and their natural disposition, natural being heavenly. This is *li*. It is difficult to translate.

Cou (腠) is even worse! On the left you have flesh, and next to it on the right you have the idea of musical rhythm, that which gives the rhythm or the beat in music. This is the idea that at each beat all the instruments will play together. When you add the water radical you have the idea of a meeting of waters, a convergence or a confluence (*cou* 湊). So in this ideogram *cou* there is the idea of a rhythmical convergence in the body. And the expression *cou li* means all the lines you see on the exterior of the body, all the ways in which the pores open and close, the way in which the natural disposition inside a being is manifest on the external surface.

Cou li is not the skin, and it is not the pores, it is something else again. Obviously all this rhythm of the skin and the pores has a very close relationship with the circulation of the defensive energy, with the different times of year and with the different times of the day. There are moments in the evening when you close down, and there are moments in the morning when things open up, just like flowers.

Claude Larre: If we follow movements in our own psychology we may think that there is a corresponding movement in the body, as if the external envelope is where the inner motion is visible. I am sure we perceive when something changes. For example when I get up in the morning I perceive the difference in my consciousness from when I was lying in bed. I can infer different phenomena taking place in my structure, and the structure is necessarily heaven and earth. So, in as much as I am a person under the influence of heaven, something is sent to me to put me into a new state of mind. But at the same time, since this heavenly inspiration has to take place somewhere, it takes place in my bodily constitution, my earthly condition. Everything on earth is visible, just as in the body *nei wai* (內 外) and *biao li* (表 裡) are always making the inner manifest to the external. So if we know what *cou li* has to express then we can understand what *cou li* might be.

Elisabeth Rochat: The internal structure of a living being can be the five *zang* and the six *fu*, and you know that the triple heater is like a link and an envelope for all these internal functions. But it is not only this, it is also the thing which contains and diffuses all the effects of this internal structure, and it is because of this that its influence goes right up to the *cou li*. The whole work of the nutritive and defensive energies is the distribution of the original *qi*, the reconstitution of the *qi*, the distribution of that which nourishes, constructs, builds and defends, and makes the movement of opening and closing the pores. Of course, there has to be the presence of the liquids produced by the middle heater, regulated by the lower heater and distributed by the upper heater, and since the bladder has a specific function on the *jin ye*, and has the quality of *qi* of *tai yang* which go right up to the most external part of the body, these naturally join with those of the triple heater in the particular resonance of their activity at the level of the *cou li.*

In a way there is no difference between the lines drawn on the skin and the rhythm of opening and closing. Both express the ultimate development and expression of my original nature in the depths.

NAN JING TEXTS

NAN JING DIFFICULTY 8

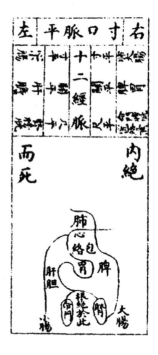

The 12 meridians all connect with the source, yuan (原), of the qi of life. What is called the source of the qi of life is the root and foundation of the 12 meridians, that is to say the qi that moves between the kidneys. These are

the foundation of the five zang and six fu, the root of the 12 meridians, the door of expiration and inspiration, the source of the three heaters. They are called the guardians of the spirits against perverse influences. Thus this qi is the root and foundation of man. When the root is exhausted, then the stem and leaves dry up. When the mai, the pulse just below the thumb, is balanced and there is death, it is because the qi is exhausted on the inside.

Elisabeth Rochat: This is someone who dies in good health. It happens to certain people. In this case there is no particular illness, there is simply an exhaustion in the *qi* of life, and this can be traced back to *ming men* (命 門), which is the source of the *qi* of life, where the meridians are connected. *Ming men* is the *qi* that moves between the two kidneys, and this forms an interesting parallel with the *qi* that moves between the two breasts, the sea of *qi*, which is the source of *zong qi* (宗 氣), the *qi* of posterior heaven, and of diffusion throughout the whole organism. But no function in the body can exist if it is not a development of the origin of life and *ming men*.

The passage continues by saying that it is the door of expiration and inspiration. The entry and exit of *qi* is not just made by the lung, but also by the triple heater and through the relationship of the lung with the kidneys. It is necessary to have the basic power of the kidneys to attract and draw the *qi* down to the deepest point in the body. In clinical practice you might see the application of this, for example in cases of asthma where one of the most important things to determine is whether the difficulty is with exhalation or inhalation. If the problem is more with exhalation the treatment will be more to do with the lung, but if it is more with inhalation then you will tonify the kidneys. Breathing in Chinese medicine is, of course, governed by the lung, under the activity of the ancestral *qi,* (*zong qi* 宗 氣), but it is rooted in the kidneys and in the lower heater because the first opening is at *ming men.*

This passage also says that the *qi* which moves between the kidneys is the source of the three heaters. What is interesting here is this word source (*yuan* 原), which is the same as in the source points we find on all the *yang* meridians. Then we also have the relationship of the triple heater with the rooting of the five *zang* and six *fu.* This can evoke the *chong mai* (衝 脈) which is the sea of the 12 meridians. So here is the connection of the triple heater with a third sea, in the form of *ming men,* or *chong mai.*

We can speculate as to whether the triple heater also has a relationship with the fourth sea, the sea of marrow, the brain. We can say that the triple heater is everywhere, and that the meridian of the triple heater penetrates the middle of the ear. We also know that the interior of the ear or eye are the means of communicating deeply with the brain. And we have the *jing bie* (經 別) or meridian divergences. The one related to the triple heater, the *shao yang* of the hand, is called 'pointer to heaven'. It detaches at the highest point of the skull in order to later go to Stomach 12. The triple heater meridian itself does not go to the top of the head, but the bladder does, so it is as if there is a delegation from the triple heater there. But this is all that I have found on this possible communication between the triple heater and the fourth sea, and it is just speculation.

Difficulty 8 continues:

> *They are called the guardians of the spirits against perverse influences.*

This is to say they are really the protection for life, and the protection of the spirits. This protection comes about by the diffusion of the power of *ming men* (命 門) and the *qi* between the kidneys, and, of course, through the activity of the triple heater. If this activity fails, the defence against perverse influences weakens and you get every sort of illness. But if it is the root itself which is exhausted, then all the effects will wither and fade. Little by little the vitality will be retracted and disappear, up to the point of death. This kind of disappearance of the triple heater, of all the functions of the *zang* and *fu*, of the meridians, and of breathing, mean it is death by means of the exhaustion of the *qi* of life, it is the end of your mandate, the end of your destiny.

NAN JING DIFFICULTY 31

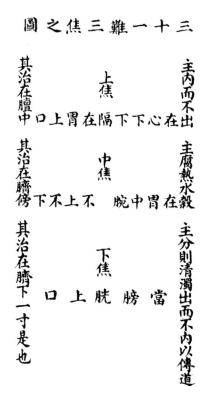

What do the three heaters receive? What do they produce?
What is their beginning and what their end? Where are
they normally treated? Is it possible to know this?

The three heaters are the ways and pathways of the liquids and cereals, the beginning and ending of the qi.

The upper heater is below the heart and descends to the diaphragm. It is at the upper mouth of the stomach. It governs the entries so that nothing goes back out. Its treatment is at tan zhong (膻 中 Ren 17), 1.6 cun below yu tang (玉 堂 Ren 18), in the hollow that is located directly between the breasts. The middle heater is located in the central cavity of the stomach, neither above nor below. It governs the rotting and cooking of the liquids and cereals. Its treatment is at the sides of the navel (possibly Stomach 25). The lower heater is at the level of the upper mouth of the bladder. It governs the division and separation of the clear and the unclear. It governs the exits so that nothing (re-)enters. Its function is transit (transporting, transmission). Its treatment is one cun below the navel (Ren 7). This is why their name is the three heaters. Their fu is at the Road of the Qi, qi jie (氣 街), or Impetuous Current of Qi, qi chong (氣 衝).

Elisabeth Rochat: *Qi chong* is the name of Stomach 30. Road of the *qi* is also all the pathways of *qi*, at the chest, on the legs, on the trunk and so on. There are, of course, four roads into the body for the distribution and circulation of all the *qi*, and they are in relationship with the triple heater. So this presentation summarizes all that we have said so far.

NAN JING DIFFICULTY 66

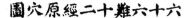

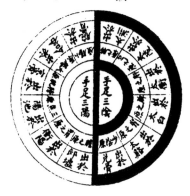

Elisabeth Rochat: The first part of this difficulty consists of a reminder about the source points of the 12 meridians, and it says that the source of the heart meridian comes out, or appears, at *da ling* (大 陵), which is the seventh point on *xin zhu* (心 主). A little further on it says that the source of the *shao yin* comes out at the slightly pointed bone, which is a way of indicating the point *shen men* (神門), Heart 7. But contrary to all the other points this one is not given a name, just a location. So here difficulty 66 presents a grouping of all 12 source points, one for each meridian. Then it says that for the *yin* meridians the *yu* (俞) points also serve as source points, and that the *yang* meridians have both a *yu* point and a *yuan* (原) point.

> *The yu of the five zang, it is there that the three heaters circulate, there where the qi resides and stops. The yu where the three heaters circulate are the sources, yuan. How is this?*

> *The qi that moves between the kidneys and under the navel - this is the life received by man. It is the root and foundation of the 12 meridians. It is for this reason that its name is source, yuan (原). The three heaters are the agents for the distribution of original qi. They govern the free circulation for the three types of qi. They rule the successive passages to the five zang and six fu. Source, yuan, is the honoured title of the three heaters. Thus where they have their own ways, that is the source. When the five zang and six fu have illnesses, one needles the source.*

Elisabeth Rochat: This is connected with what is said in Nan jing difficulty 62, which specifically talks about the source points on the *yang* meridians.

NAN JING DIFFICULTY 62

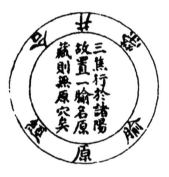

The zang have five in the series jing (井), *rong* (榮) *[etc],*
but the fu have six. How is this?

It is because the fu are yang. For its circulation linked
with all the yang it is necessary for the three heaters to
have a yu whose name is yuan. But the fu have six of
them and with the three heaters they unite in a single
breath.

Elisabeth Rochat: These two difficulties, 62 and 66, put the source points in relationship with the triple heater. The triple heater takes its source in the original *qi* of *ming men* (命 門), and is the intermediary between *ming men* and all the functions of the body which need the constant presence of the original *qi*. It is their agent or messenger. As the text of difficulty 66 says:

> *The three heaters are the agents for the distribution of original qi, yuan qi zhi bie shi* (元 氣 之 別 使).

Yuan qi (元 氣) means the original *qi*, *bie* (別) means detached, and *shi* (使) is the servant, the ambassador, or the agent, the messenger: the agent for the detachment (and distribution) of original *qi*. So this is what the triple heater represents for the original *qi*, it remains attached to the source but goes everywhere to activate things like a servant. It acts to produce all the effects that this *qi* commands in every place in the organism. This being done, all free communication and circulation goes well, and in particular the circulation of what we call the three types of *qi*, which we can consider as being the ancestral, nutritive and defensive - each of them attached to one of the three heaters. But we can also think of it as the expression of the original, unique and single breath in all its possible diversification. All this is marked by the number three, which is the number of *qi* and the number for animation.

This original *qi,* through the intermediary of the triple heater, crosses and impregnates the five *zang* and six *fu.* The triple heater is a way of naming this relation and communication with the origin, and for this reason each function will have a specific place where we can reinforce it. These places are what we call the source points. It is for this reason that the triple heater has a direct relationship with the source points because they are nothing except a reminder of the link with the origin. This is why in difficulty 66 it says that when the five *zang* and six *fu* are ill you needle the source.

It is also interesting to see that there is a difference between the *yin* and *yang* meridians. For the *yin* meridians this point where you once again make contact with the origin is also the *yu* (俞) point, but the *yu* point on *yin* meridians is also the point that corresponds with the earth element, and it is in the earth element par excellence that the five *zang* find their source. The five *zang* are regulated on the *yin* model, and their equilibrium is founded on the image of the five elements on the earth. On the other hand the six *fu* and the *yang* meridians which correspond with them are regulated above all by *yang,* and they echo the six *qi* of heaven, and model themselves on this. They are also the six means of joining the *qi* of heaven and earth, and for this reason points other than those marking the five elements are chosen on the *yang* meridians to show their specific rooting in this sixth *qi* of heaven, in this fire which is actually represented and diffused by the triple heater.

When it says in Nan jing difficulty 62 that 'the fu have six of them and with the three heaters they unite in a single breath' it means that the triple heater, although it is the agent of distribution, is detached, multiplies and is omnipresent, and directs all the different sorts of *qi* in the organism, through its rooting in the original *qi* is also always the representation of this unity, and this is marked by the sixth point on the *yang* meridians. This is an explanation of the source points as it is given in the Nan jing, along with the very close relationship with everything that we call the triple heater, which has a name but no form. It has no form because it is the intermediary between that which has no form and that which is formulated and becomes a form. My personal feeling is that the triple heater does not exist until after the first breath is taken, although this is never spoken about in the texts.

Claude Larre: We see again the question of who is giving life to whom? If the mother is giving life to the baby then we can see why the mother is able to do what she is supposed to do through the triple heater. It is very difficult to see the mother and child separated when the child is connected with the mother. After the birth something is needed to be the intermediary between the original *qi* (*yuan qi* 元 氣), and all the functions of life.

Elisabeth Rochat: The triple heater acts in the best possible way to ensure free communication and circulation, but the fact that everything can communicate is due to the original unity.

HUA TUO

We will finish with a translation of the text attributed to Hua Tuo from the 2nd or 3rd centry AD, although in fact the text was written much later in the Song dynasty.

> *The triple heater - the qi of the triple origin of man. When the triple heater ensures free communication, then there is free communication internally and externally, left and right, above and below. The whole body is irrigated, harmonized internally and regulated externally, nourished by the left, and maintained by the right, directed from above, propagated from below. There is nothing greater!*

SUN SIMIAO

There is another text from Sun Simiao in the 8th century. He was a very great acupuncturist and specialist in herbal medicine in the Tang dynasty. He says:

> *The three heaters through their reunion make the unity.*

They govern the way of the spirits (shen dao 神 道), which come and go in the five zang and six fu. They know how to distribute life in the form of qi, they are connected to the origin, they make the blood and maintain life through the spirits.

So there is no limit to this kind of total encompassing quality of the triple heater. It crosses throughout the body making different circuits, and this means that the triple heater has no distinct form. One can feel it, and have a certain knowledge of it, but you cannot see it. It creates the harmony and proper functioning of the essences and *qi*. It opens the passages and ensures free communication. Through blood and *qi* it allows life to continue - thanks to the spirits.

Claude Larre: My final word would be that the three heaters are seen in front of you. The first is Elisabeth who is heavily spirited, the middle one is Peter, and the third is myself!

Elisabeth Rochat: But you are the original fire!

Claude Larre: And what is done here is the warming of the general atmosphere, because I myself feel that in friendship mixed with knowledge we make the heating system we need for better acupuncture.

APPENDIX

A SUMMARY OF THE TRIPLE HEATER

E. Rochat de la Vallée and M. Macé

San jiao (三 焦), the triple heater, is one of the most difficult concepts to grasp in Chinese medicine, not only because as an entity it has no equivalent in Western medicine, but also because in China itself it has not been clearly and plainly defined.

In fact the triple heater can be presented equally as a concrete and localised organ, such as the pipes for evacuating urine or the cavities of the stomach, or as very general functions for the animation and irrigation of the whole body. The triple heater appears in the texts of the Nei jing as one of the six *fu* with the stomach, the two intestines, the bladder and the gallbladder. With the exception of the gallbladder, (Su wen 11) they form the set of *fu* for transmission and transformation, *chuan hua zhi fu* (傳 化 之 府), in charge of digestion, assimilation and elimination.

Although several texts in the Nei jing give glimpses of the regions that are under the authority of each of the heaters, it is the Nan jing 31 that clarifies their positions. The upper heater encompasses the chest, the middle heater the stomach cavity, and the lower heater the area of evacuation below. The heart and lungs are associated with the upper heater, the spleen and stomach with the middle heater, and the kidneys, intestines and bladder with the lower heater. The liver, along with the gallbladder, is usually linked to the lower heater, although certain interpretations place it with the functions of the middle heater.

The triple heater is sometimes specifically linked to the kidneys (Ling shu 2 and 47) forming one of the two *fu* corrresponding to the *zang* of the kidneys (with the bladder). It is certainly through this link with the kidneys that it fulfils the charge of opening passages and irrigating talked about in Su wen 8, thus allowing the proper management of liquids in the body. The link with the transformation of liquids is constantly confirmed in its pathology, as its relationship with water, in all its forms, is emphasised by the traditional titles attributed to each of the three heaters (Ling shu 18):

•*Wu* (霧), mist or humid vapours for the upper heater

• *Ou* (漚), maceration for the middle heater

• *Du* (瀆), canal or conduit for the lower heater

The triple heater plays a role in all stages of digestion and assimilation. It regulates the body fluids and their distribution. The fire inherent in its character was seen to play an increasingly important role in the activity of each of its three parts. In the Ming dynasty, for example in the Yixue Shengshuan of Yu Tuan, it was considered that the triple heater was the fire that circulated in the median to develop all life, the minister fire, the element to which the triple heater is linked.

Nan jing difficulty 66 presents the triple heater as the agent of distribution of original *qi* and gives it the title of *yuan*, origin. It is through the same theory that the Nan jing difficulty 62 gives the triple heater as responsible for the power of the *yuan* (原), source, points on the *yang* meridians.

One can then easily link to the three levels of the triple heater the three fundamental *qi* of life that constantly regenerate man:

• the ancestral *qi* (宗 氣 *zong qi*) in the upper heater

• the nutritive *qi* (營 氣 *ying qi*) in the middle heater

• the defensive *qi* (衛 氣 *wei qi*) in the lower heater

The defensive *qi* is related to the lower heater even though for its distribution in the body, the defensive *qi* leaves through the distributive movement proper to the lung, the sea of *qi* in the chest, in the upper heater. This mixing of fire and water that is characteristic of the triple heater recalls the joining of *yin yang* at the origin of a being's life.

Thus, the relationship of the triple heater with the origin of life in man developed in parallel with the concept of *ming men* and with reflections on the origin of all the organic constituents of life in man through water and the original fire, the authentic *yin* and *yang*, dependent on the kidneys and *ming men* (命 門).

Its double fire-water polarity makes it the representative of the origin of life, which diversifies and persists at the heart of transformations. The triple heater was increasingly linked with the notion of transformation through the work of the *qi, qi hua* (氣 化). Wang Shuhe in the Mai jing put the triple heater in a *biao li* (表 裡) relationship with *ming men*, while it is more usually coupled with the *xin bao luo* (心 包 絡) (Nan jing 25, Ling shu 10). But in either case, the couple represents the functions of minister fire, *xiang huo* (相 火), in the body. In the Tang dynasty, Sun Simiao emphasised its ability to unify all the elements of the body (Qianjin fang). The triple heater gathers together all the *zang* and *fu* and allows them to function in unity.

This unity is fully expressed in the texts of the Song dynasty (Zhongzang jing of the alleged Hua tuo) or the Yuan dynasty (Dongyuan shishu of Li Gao) where the three heaters incorporate all the functions and circulations of the body, and extend from the top of the head to the heart (upper heater), from the heart to the navel (middle heater), and from the navel to the feet (lower heater).

They are then truly considered as the triple origin in man, the final development and theorisation of what was begun in the Nan jing through their double fire-water polarity (Nan jing difficulty 31) and link with the original *qi* (Nan jing difficulties 8, 62 and 66). Function conclusively supplanted localization or purely anatomical definition: they have a name but not a form (Nan jing difficulties 25, 38). The unified *qi* of the body with its different functions and varied intensity circulates everywhere. This *qi* drives the liquids and the vital nourishing elements, allowing the transformations through which the *qi* and essences are renewed and by which the organs function. The union of *qi* and water, at work in these vital mechanisms, is well represented by the triple heater (Ling shu 36, Nan jing difficulty 31 etc). This does not limit it from being the simple reunion of the organs located in each of the levels, but in a more far-reaching way it represents the synergy of all the *zang fu*, renewing and properly circulating *qi* and liquids without stagnation or shortage.

INDEX